# The Wondrous World of Social Dancing in Canada

### Come Dance Ballroom, Salsa, Square-dance and Argentine Tango with Me!

## JOHN YUEN

The Wondrous World of Social Dancing in Canada: Come Dance Ballroom, Salsa, Square-dance and Argentine Tango with Me!

Copyright 2021 by John Yuen
All rights reserved.

ISBN 978-1-7777146-0-4

Cover design by Laura Boyle
Interior design by Woven Red Author Services, www.WovenRed.ca

Published by Simcoe Publishing
P.O. Box 64
Georgina, Ontario
L4P 3E1
Email: info@simcoepublishing.ca
https://simcoepublishing.ca/
*The Wondrous World of Social Dancing in Canada*
John Yuen

Back cover photos: Mandy Epprecht, (Ray Vella, Mississauga,, ON, www.rvphotos.ca/ Magdalena Rudzik, (M. Rudzik); Nina & Anuj Chandarana (N. Chandarana); Doug & Gayle Allen (Doug Allen); Bert & Shirley Lajoie (Shirley Lajoie);and Martina & Lorne (M.Sommer).

For Jeff Henssen and all the instructors who have taught me all that I know about good social dancing, and for my students from whom I have learned a lot.

# Contents

Figures ........................................................................................................... 13

About Social Dancing ................................................................................... 15

Foreword ....................................................................................................... 17

Preface .......................................................................................................... 21

Acknowledgements ....................................................................................... 23

Introduction .................................................................................................. 25

**Chapter 1, Part 1: Up to the 17th Century** ................................................ 31
    Inuit, Métis, And Other First Peoples ...................................................... 31
        Inuvialuit Dancing ............................................................................. 32
        Métis Dancing .................................................................................... 32
    Canada's First Settlers and Dancing in New France ................................. 35
        The First Social Club Is Set Up .......................................................... 37
        Dancing Was the Colonists' Top Hobby ........................................... 38

**Chapter 1, Part 2: The 18th and 19th Centuries** ....................................... 42
    18th Century Canada: People, Economy, and Social Dancing ................. 42
        The Most Popular Ballroom Dances ................................................. 43
    19th Century Canada: People, Economy, And Social Dancing ................ 44
        Technology Spreads the Popularity of Dancing ................................ 46
        Following the Rules of the Dancing Game ....................................... 49
        The State and Churches: Opposition to Dancing ............................. 52
        Prince Charles Dancing with the Locals: The 1860 Royal Tour ........ 55
        Dining, Drinking, and Dancing Close to Confederation (1867) ........ 56
        Dancing After Confederation (1867) ................................................. 58

**Chapter 1, Part 3: 20th Century to the Present** ....................................... 62
    20th Century Canada: People, Economy and Social Dancing Life ......... 62
    From the 1900s until the Second World War ........................................... 63
        Latin Dances Appear ......................................................................... 66
        Montréal Develops a Reputation for Jazz Nights ............................. 69

- Ballroom Dances and the Dance Industry in the 1920s ... 70
- 1940s to 1960s: Good Dancing Times for Urban Masses ... 71
  - Drinking and Dancing ... 76
- From 1960s to 2020s: Growing and Maturing ... 77
  - Public Funding for Training Young Bodies and Minds for Dancing ... 77
  - Arrival of Eastern European Immigrant Dancers ... 79
  - The 2014 Canada Dance Mapping Study ... 79
  - The New Ballroom Style ... 80
  - Social Dancing Becomes Popular Again Then Dips ... 82
  - The COVID-19 Pandemic: Tales of Hope for Social Dancers ... 84
  - The National Square and Round Dance Community ... 86
  - Nunavut ... 86
  - British Columbia ... 87
  - **A**lberta ... 87
  - Saskatchewan ... 87
  - Manitoba ... 88
  - Ontario ... 88
  - Québec ... 89
  - New Brunswick ... 90
  - Nova Scotia ... 90
- Conclusion ... 91

## Chapter 2: Having the Time of Their Social Dancing Life! ... 96
- Living and Dancing ... 96
- Social Dancers' Thoughts on Their Passion and Art ... 99
- What It Really Means ... 99
  - Ying Cheung in Vancouver and social ballroom/Latin ... 99
  - Vivian Brailean in Moose Jaw, Saskatchewan, and square dancing ... 100
  - Dorothy Campbell and partner in Saskatoon, Saskatchewan. and square dancing ... 100
  - Nella and Patrick Keating in Bradford-West Gwillimbury, Ontario, and social ballroom/Latin ... 103
  - Eleanor Dyke and Dean Little in Bradford-West Gwillimbury and social ballroom/Latin ... 103
  - Jeanette and John Kanyo in Bradford-West Gwillimbury and social ballroom/Latin ... 103
  - Dale and J.J. Lubberts in East Gwillimbury, Ontario, and social ballroom/Latin ... 104
  - Jacinta Willems in Mitchell, Ontario, and Argentine tango ... 104
  - Karen Paton-Evans and Jim Evans in Shakespeare, Ontario, and social ballroom/Latin ... 105

Maria Dobrynina and Alex Dobrynin in Newmarket, Ontario, and social ballroom/Latin ..................................................................................................105
Diane Ternan and David Franks in Newmarket and social ballroom/Latin ...........................................................................................................................106
Sandra Holliday-Tucker and Silas ("Sie") Tucker in Newmarket and social ballroom/Latin ..................................................................................................106
Liboire (a.k.a. Lee) Brossard in Montréal and salsa ............................................107
Esther and Barry Stanfield in Saint-Bruno, Québec and square dancing 107
Cristina Chirca in Montréal and salsa ..................................................................107
Kathryn Stone in Halifax, Nova Scotia and Argentine tango ........................ 108
Vaunda and Martin Vanderaa in Charlottetown, Prince Edward Island, and square dancing ............................................................................................ 108

## Getting Started on the Journey .................................................................108
Merv Meyer in Kamloops, British Columbia, and square dancing ................ 108
Vivian Brailean in Moose Jaw, Saskatchewan, and square dancing ............109
Dale and J.J. Lubberts in East Gwillimbury and social ballroom/Latin ......109
Dianne and Dominic Panacci in King, Ontario, and social ballroom/Latin 110
Nina Chandarana in Toronto and salsa ................................................................110
Patricia Lam in Toronto and Argentine tango ....................................................110
Minoo Asgary and Omar Kazi in Toronto and Argentine tango ..................... 111
Pat Mastrandrea in Newmarket, Ontario, and social ballroom/Latin .......... 111
Hindy Borstein in Richmond Hill, Ontario, and "Olde Tyme" square dancing ............................................................................................................................112
Nina Chandarana in Toronto and salsa ................................................................112
Santha and Ivan Leong in Toronto and social ballroom/Latin ...................... 113
Liboire (a.k.a. Lee) Brossard in Montréal and salsa .......................................... 113
Cristina Chirca in Montréal and salsa .................................................................. 113
Vahide Morina in Halifax, Nova Scotia and salsa ............................................. 114
Marg and Larry Clark in Halifax and Argentine tango ................................... 114
Carla Anglehart in Halifax and Argentine tango ............................................. 114
Alexander Carleton in Fredericton, New Brunswick and swing ................... 115
Kathryn Stone in Halifax, Nova Scotia and Argentine tango ........................ 115

## Instructors' Guidance on the Ground ........................................................116
Louise McKay and Tadahiro Okazawa in Calgary and Argentine tango ..... 116
Karen Paton-Evans and Jim Evans in Shakespeare, Ontario, and social ballroom/Latin ................................................................................................... 116
Jacinta Willems in Mitchell, Ontario, and Argentine tango ............................117
John Loomis in Mississauga and Argentine tango ............................................117
Andria W. in Toronto and social ballroom/Latin ...............................................117
Minoo Asgary and Omar Kazi in Toronto and Argentine tango .................... 118
Cindy Stradling and Lino in Toronto and social ballroom/Latin ................... 118
Liboire (a.k.a. Lee) Brossard in Montréal and salsa .......................................... 119

- Practising the Moves........................................................................................... 119
  - Diane Ternan and David Franks in Newmarket, Ontario and social ballroom/Latin............................................................................................ 119
  - Santha and Ivan Leong in Markham, Ontario and social ballroom/Latin. 120
  - Monika Szymczak in Toronto and social ballroom/Latin........................ 120
  - Patricia Lam in Toronto and Argentine tango ........................................ 120
  - Jacinta Willems in Mitchell, Ontario and Argentine tango ..................... 121
  - Pat Mastrandrea in Newmarket, Ontario, and social ballroom/Latin...... 121
  - Cindy Stradling in Toronto and social ballroom/Latin ........................... 121
  - Andria W. in Toronto and social ballroom/Latin .................................... 122
  - Vahide Morina in Halifax and salsa ......................................................... 122
  - Alexander Carleton in Fredericton, New Brunswick and swing.............. 122
  - Cristina Chirca in Montréal and salsa ..................................................... 123
- Most Enjoyable Moments Dancing.................................................................... 123
  - Timothy Tan in Vancouver and social ballroom/Latin............................. 123
  - Arkady Silverman in Toronto and social ballroom/Latin......................... 123
  - Alice Meinecke in Bracebridge, Ontario, and square dancing................ 124
  - Sandra Holliday-Tucker and Silas ("Sie") Tucker in Newmarket and social ballroom/Latin................................................................................ 124
  - Nina Chandarana in Toronto and salsa................................................... 124
  - Monika Szymczak in Toronto and social ballroom/Latin........................ 125
  - Karen Paton-Evans and Jim Evans in Shakespeare, Ontario, and social ballroom/Latin............................................................................................ 125
  - Patricia Lam in Toronto and Argentine tango ........................................ 125
  - Liboire (a.k.a. Lee) Brossard in Montréal and salsa................................ 125
  - Vahide Morina in Halifax, Nova Scotia and salsa.................................... 126
  - Marg and Larry Clark in Halifax and Argentine tango ........................... 126
  - Carla Anglehart in Halifax and Argentine tango..................................... 126
  - Vaunda and Martin Vanderaa in Charlottetown, Prince Edward Island and square dancing ..................................................................................... 127
- Conclusion........................................................................................................... 127

# Chapter 3: Joyful Moments for Special Dancers............................................ 129
- Wheelchair-Bound Dancers............................................................................... 130
- Organizations Pitch In ....................................................................................... 132
- Various Dance Forms for Dancers with Disabilities ........................................ 134
- Argentine Tango, a Boon to the Life of Two Nova Scotia Dancers with PD ................................................................................................................ 135
- Conclusion........................................................................................................... 136

## Chapter 4: The Dance Academy—Watching Over Dancers Each Step of the Way ... 138

### The Ballroom/Latin Academy ... 140
- Seasoned Practitioners Lead the Pack ... 140
- Diverse Teachers in Social Ballroom/Latin ... 141

### The Salsa Dance Academy ... 143
- Diverse Teachers in Salsa ... 145

### The Argentine Tango Dance Academy ... 149
- Diverse Teachers in Argentine Tango ... 150

### The Volunteer-based Square Dance and Round Dance Academy ... 151
- Olde Tyme Square Dancing and Modern Square Dancing ... 153
- Facing the Future—Two National Square Dance Associations ... 154

### Municipal 'Leisure Services'—A Social Dance Academy ... 155

### Author's 2018-2019 Survey of Social Dance Classes ... 156
- Overall Response ... 156
- The Questions ... 156
- Details of Responses ... 156
- Commentary on the Demographics of Participants During 2018-2019 .. 158
- Experience in Providing Dance Services ... 160

### Indie Instructors at Volunteer-run Dance Clubs ... 163

### 'Helping Out' the Social Clubs ... 164

### Conclusion ... 164

## Appendix A: "The 39 Opinions" on competitive dancing, a representation of social dance ... 167

## Appendix B: Select list of Canadian Social Dance Academies by Province /Territory and Four Dance Forms ... 173

### Argentine Tango ... 173
- Alberta ... 173
- British Columbia ... 174
- Manitoba ... 175
- New Brunswick, Newfoundland & Labrador ... 175
- Nova Scotia ... 175
- Ontario ... 175
- Prince Edward Island ... 177
- Québec ... 177
- Saskatchewan ... 177

### Ballroom/Latin ... 178
- Alberta ... 178

    British Columbia .......... 179
    Manitoba .......... 180
    New Brunswick .......... 180
    Newfoundland and Labrador .......... 180
    Nova Scotia .......... 181
    Ontario .......... 181
    Prince Edward Island .......... 186
    Quebéc .......... 187
    Saskatchewan .......... 187
Salsa .......... 188
    Alberta .......... 188
    British Columbia .......... 188
    Manitoba .......... 190
    New Brunswick .......... 190
    Newfoundland & Labrador .......... 190
    Nova Scotia .......... 190
    Ontario .......... 191
    Prince Edward Island .......... 194
    Québec .......... 194
    Saskatchewan .......... 195
Square Dancing .......... 195
    Alberta .......... 195
    British Columbia .......... 197
    Manitoba .......... 199
    New Brunswick .......... 199
Newfoundland & Labrador .......... 200
    Nova Scotia .......... 200
    Ontario .......... 201
    Prince Edward Island .......... 203
    Quebéc .......... 203
    Saskatchewan .......... 203
Round Dancing .......... 204
    Alberta .......... 204
    British Columbia .......... 204
    Ontario .......... 204
    Manitoba .......... 205
    New Brunswick .......... 205
    Newfoundland & Labrador .......... 205
    Nova Scotia .......... 205
    Prince Edward Island .......... 205
    Quebéc .......... 205

    Saskatchewan...................................................................................205

About the Author..........................................................................207

References....................................................................................209
    Telephone Interviews........................................................209
    Correspondence from Individuals....................................211
    Correspondence from Organizations ...............................211

Bibliography ................................................................................213
    Mass Media.........................................................................224
    Social Media.......................................................................224

Index.............................................................................................225

# Figures

(Photo courtesy in parentheses/italics.)

1. Fairmont Royal York Hotel today (formerly Royal York) in Toronto. Chapter 1. *(John Yuen)*.
2. The Matador Building Chapter 1. *(J. Yuen)*
3. Six ballroom dancers in Bradford West Gwillimbury. Chapter 2. *(Eleanor Dyke)*.
4. B.C. Latin dancers Timothy Tan and Theresa Bodnarchuk, Chapter 2. *(Timothy Tan and UBC Dance Club)*.
5. Toronto's Minoo Asgar and Omar Kazi dressed up for dancing, Chapter 2. *(Minoo Asgar)*.
6. Sitting dancers outdoors and indoors. Chapter 3. Outdoor photo, *(unknown)*, indoor photo, *(Robert Straight)*.
7. Brenton Mitchell & Jane Edgett, Chapter 4. *(B. Mitchell)*.
8. Aleks Saiyan, Chapter 4. *(A. Saiyan)*.
9. Leo Sato, Chapter 4 ((*L. Sato)*.
10. Square dance caller Linda Gilchrist, Chapter 4. *(L. Gilchrist)*.
11. Andy & Wendy Wong, Chapter 4 *(A.Wong)*
12. Sandra Campanelli, Chapter 4 *(S. Campanelli)*

# About Social Dancing

- ❖ Social dancing is pursued for play and pleasure.
- ❖ It can be done solo, with a partner or as a group, with or without music.
- ❖ A huge swath of Canada's 38 million residents, from all walks of life, have danced socially at one time or another.
- ❖ For Indigenous people, music and dance are part of their everyday life.
- ❖ Competitive dancing, such as dancesport and salsa competitions, is not social dance but is a representation of it.
- ❖ This book covers four of the most popular social dances Canadians pursue.

# Foreword

For the first time, here is a comprehensive, detailed study of the historical development of modern social dancing in Canada, and how the development of North American culture has influenced dance throughout the past five hundred years.

John Yuen brings his many years of experience as a journalist and dance teacher, to delve deep into the social, ceremonial and spiritual aspects of Canada's history of social dance. He begins with the Indigenous community from the seventeenth century, through the arrival of centuries-old dances brought to Canada by European and American settlers, and finally to our current times and the rapidly increasing popularity of salsa, Argentine tango, social ballroom/Latin and modern square dancing.

This fascinating study brings to life the many ways dance has changed and adapted throughout our history. It explores what aspects of life, such as fashion or technological improvements, have influenced the development of social dance, and what an important role it has played in Canadian culture.

This is a captivating look at how modern ballroom dance has become standardized, how it has changed from being a mostly upper-class activity, to being integrated into mainstream society, and how it has become an integral part of modern society.

There are plenty of references from experts from all over the world who offer personal and interesting insights into the many uplifting experiences that social dance brings, as well as testimonials from all levels of dance enthusiasts from across Canada.

Bringing the story of dance into modern times, the author details the devastating effects of the COVID-19 pandemic which has brought dancing throughout the world to a standstill. Interviews with highly qualified and respected dance teachers from across the country offer insight into how it will affect the social dance scene, and how it will recover.

This is a joyful book, filled with fascinating historical details, as well as an in depth look at the therapeutic benefits of dance. The final chapter is an intriguing look at the who's, what's, and why's of becoming a dance teacher in Canada, and includes the most comprehensive list of schools, clubs and teachers across the country that has ever been collected.

Here you will find an in-depth study of dance in Canada, expertly written, for dancers or non-dancers alike.

Mandy Epprecht
Owner
*Mandy's Dance*
Mississauga, ON

Dance—it's within us all. The unmistakable and undeniable physical reaction that we, human beings, have to music. It is a connection, a relationship to something outside of oneself.

Social dancing takes it one step further. While dancing together on a current of music, social dancers give and take, respect and acknowledge each other, listen and respond and thus are connected to their partners in that not-to-be repeated moment and space in time. Even one step further, they are connected to the other dancers on the floor by their practice of navigation, their awareness, acknowledgement of and respect for their surroundings; for their surrounding fellow dancers who are, for that moment teammates if you will, dancing to the same melody.

And so, one of the fundamental human needs and traits—that of attachment—is played out in a multitude of ways on the social dance floor. No wonder it feels so good, is so satisfying and provides so many proven benefits to its many practitioners!

(All this without even mentioning all the fun stuff such as great music, new friends, exercise, weight loss, improved core strength and balance, improved mental acuity, dressing up, going to dance parties and just plain old having the confidence to step onto the dance floor!)

In this book, John Yuen paints a lively picture of what social dancing has meant and continues to mean to people in Canada. It is delightful to discover how similar are the sentiments of present-day dancers to those expressed by dancers from a hundred and fifty years ago. Presumably, similar thoughts will be expressed by future dancers: Perhaps you?

Not only does the author demonstrate the importance of social dance to the individual but also how it ties into the economic and diverse cultural Canadian community. He talks about the various small and big institutions involved in social dance giving the reader ideas of what to expect when going out dancing, what to look for in an instructor and where to go to learn to dance. From his very thoroughly researched anecdotes of dancing in the past to his interviews with modern-day dancers from all walks of life, it is definitive—social dancing matters.

During my twenty-five years in this industry as a student, competitor, instructor and studio owner, I have witnessed time and again how dancers leave the dance floor in a better state than when they first stepped onto it.

With the prevailing topic of mental well-being in the news, social dancing might just be, if not quite a panacea, then at least a part of the answer to what everyone is looking for. And I believe firmly that if more people danced socially, the world would be a better place.

Let this book intrigue you. If you are a dancer, you will find kinship with fellow dancers whose thoughts are present in this text and if you are not yet a dancer, this book might just convince you to give it a try. Then you can go forth and dance, and make this world a better place, one "step" (pun intended) at a time!

Magdalena Rudzik<br>
Studio Director<br>
*Dancing for Dessert Studio*<br>
Langley, B.C.

# Preface

I can clearly remember standing in a long line with other men of various ages opposite a line of women, both young and older, ready to hear the social dance instructor's prompt, "OK, take a partner!"

The next thing me and the other men were supposed to do was to quickly ask the nearest lady—or "the one you secretly admire"—to practise the figures for dances such as quickstep, slow waltz, rumba and cha-cha-cha.

This happened a lot for me during the 1980s in dimly lit dance halls in Toronto, where I spent most of my life. At the time, I had "two left feet," so to speak. But each week I was able to better command the movements of my head, hips and hands—and feet, of course—to.do the bidding of my instructors.

They were all truly excellent at demonstrating how to partner with someone and how to understand the music played by deejays and live orchestras.

When I look back over the many years I took classes—both group and private—I realize my teachers could have told me much more about the history of Canadian social dancing than they ever did. Hearing more of how we got here would definitely have made my learning experiences in dance so much more enjoyable.

For example, I now know—but was not aware earlier—that a century ago, the Argentine tango was a "wicked" thing to do in Montréal before Torontonians lapped it up. Or, that social ballroom dancing was a favourite pastime of several past governors general after we became a nation and that for ordinary people it was also *numero uno*.

Describing Canadians dancing in the distant past, as if talking about hockey in present-day Canada, Edwin G. Guillet of Cobourg, Ontario once wrote: "Of all the amusements of early times, dancing was the most universal and appears to have given the greatest pleasure to the greatest number."

The history of our dancing days and ways—fascinating!

And that is a big part of the reason why this book came to be.

I have enjoyed doing the primary sources research (interviewing people and locating original printed documents) as well as the secondary sources research (books and magazine articles about social dancing by Canadian and other historians).

The hundred-plus people I contacted from coast-to-coast for interviews were very friendly and open with their opinions. I was grateful for that.

It was quite a revelatory experience pulling together the remarkable credentials of instructors as well as studio/club listings for salsa, social ballroom/Latin, Argentine tango and square dancing in this country. Readers, as dance services consumers, will now have a sharper appreciation of the choices available to them and be able to make more informed decisions regarding who to go to and where.

This book only scratches the surface of what Canadians have done and are doing in the realm of social dancing. Much more needs to be brought to light by other authors who are willing to take up the challenge.

# Acknowledgements

A considerable number of people have helped me, directly or indirectly, in preparing this book.

I would like to thank the staff in Ontario's public libraries (Toronto, Aurora, Georgina), Libraries and Archives Canada, and Ryerson and York Universities for providing resources that I could not otherwise have access to. My appreciation also to Elisabeth Dobson and Amy Bowring of Dance Collection Danse in Toronto for allowing me to review their historical materials.

My gratitude to all those who made time for me to be interviewed, especially given the different time zones. They include social dancers, instructors, spokespersons for social dance organizations, and even competitive dancers and others.

The 2018-2019 survey of Canadian municipalities described in Chapter 4, would have been impossible without the cooperation of their senior administrators and other staff who worked diligently to compile statistics on those who registered for social dance classes in their facilities. They are Barb Armstrong, Scott Bisson, Darby Boyd, Parm Chohan, Claude Danis, Naomi Evans, Patricia Fillet, Donna Flatman, Faye Forbes-Anderson, Tanya Grierson, Alex Hamilton, Laura Hanna, Colleen Lichti, Jerry Jestin, Janis Luttrell, Kathy Masterson, Karen Miller, Jeremy Neill, Joey Ouellette, Marie-Pier Paquette-Séguin, LoriAnn Palubeski, Nancy Shortill-Thatcher, Maggie-Jane Spray, and Adam Viola. These persons and their associated municipalities are listed at the back of the book.

I appreciate the view of the thirty-nine persons across the country who gave me their take on competitive dancing, a representation of social dance. In the *Thirty Nine Opinions* feature titled Appendix A, readers can learn about their perspectives which are wide-ranging and may inspire those who now only dance socially, to consider going farther afield with their talents.

My good friends Francesco Pugliese, Ada Kelly and John Stefaniak provided much-appreciated input on the title.

I owe thanks to friends and colleagues in the Argentine tango, salsa, social ballroom, and the square dance sectors with whom I shared thoughts and ideas in person and electronically. My heartfelt indebtedness, therefore, to Alessandra Amaro, Giorgio Argentini, Gabia Antony, Minoo Asgar, Kathryn Baird, Halina Bodnar, Anna Borshch, Lorne Buick, Sandra Campanelli, Shirley Caron, Nina Chandarana, Frederick Chen, Juliana Chow, Laura Dawson, Rene Delgado, Cristina Amalia Dina, Eleanor Dyke, Mandy Epprecht, Leah Frei, Oleo Gonzalo, Andrea Gonsalves, Trena Graham, Susi Haemmerle, Rev. Daniel F. Graves, Gabby Holt, Ada Kelley, Ali Neen Khan, Monika Kodnani, Flori Mackie, Sylvia McKinley, Steve Nelson, Ralph Price, Magda Rudzik, Megan Walter Straight, Robert Straight, Bill Russell, Elizabeth Sadowska, Aleksander Saiyan, Leo Sato, Martina Sommer, John Stefaniak, Marjorie White, Melody Vallerand and Terry Tzee Zaifman.

My great appreciation to bilingual ballroom and Latin dancer Ginette Kanyo for help in liaising with Francophone individuals residing in Québec. My gratitude to Eleanor Dyke, Dean Little, Ginette, her husband, John Kanyo, and Francesco Pugliese for general advice on content. I am supremely grateful to proofreader Santha Leung, whose discovery of misspellings in the final draft has saved me from future embarrassments. Ultimately, however, I take full responsibility for any errors that appear.

A special thank-you to my sister, Rosemarie Foley, who took to the phone lines many times to link me up with a group of Western Canada contacts who were not only super friendly but also provided insightful views about dancing.

# Introduction

Clinton Collier, the administrator of a popular Facebook page on social dancing in Toronto, posted a picture on April 24, 2021 of Karen Abi Nader and Apo Najarian dancing bachata, a popular companion dance to salsa.

He questioned whether it was really bachata because they seemed to be "pulling in" different styles and variations. The couple was clearly improvising. Yet Karen and Apo got rave reviews on YouTube.

Improvising dance steps has been going on for years. When people go out dancing, they often forget steps they learned in classes and do just that— "pulling in" figures from the different dance forms they are learning.

That's OK. There are no dance police officers, so people can do whatever they want. Enjoying what they are doing is what matters.

What is happening now is that the Latin dances have been changing in Canada and the U.S. like they did a century ago.

During the Roaring Twenties, the ragtime dances and the "animal dances" (such as the horse trot, chicken scratch, turkey trot, and grizzly bear) went through a similar period of changes. Even nineteenth-century dances that persisted in the twentieth century were not immune to what was going on. Dancers mixed the steps over time and expressed their individuality.

The improvisation trend did not affect modern ballroom dances, because the colonial masters of ballroom dancing had set up an iron ring around them. Rules and protocols for the waltzes, quickstep, and foxtrot were in place.

This trend has taken hold here, so when people dance salsa or other Latin dances such as bachata, kizomba and zouk, they often interchange figures.

In fact, Chapter 1 of this book shows that improvising in dancing occurred a lot through Canada's social dancing history. For example, while our colonial administrators (both French and English) and the elite members of society were dancing the cotillion, minuet and gavotte, ordinary folks in the rural parts of the provinces were mimicking those dances as well as the English country dances and did them the way they wanted. They did their own thing, as the saying goes.

Other chapters of the book zoom in on the present dancing landscape.

In Chapter 2, readers will read the spontaneous words of dancers across the land regarding how they feel about being part of the social dancing world. The dancers speak from the heart and do so without being anonymous. They touch on why they dance, how they got started, what they think of their instruction, and how much commitment they give to it.

Chapter 3 is fascinating in the sense that we learn how thousands of Canadians who have physical limitations brought on by diseases or disability are enjoying various modified forms of social dances, including Argentine tango. Those who have the courage to participate in these activities discuss their success in better physical control and warding off social isolation to a great extent.

Readers will learn how major organizations such as the National Ballet of Canada, the nation-wide Parkinson Society, and Dancing for PD (an international body based in New York with multiple facilities in Canada) are providing relief for people with Parkinson's disease (PD). Through a network of dance studios from Newfoundland to British Columbia, thousands of people with PD access specific techniques and methods to improve balance, flexibility, and strength through music and movement using social dances.

Even smaller organizations such as the Nova Scotia-based *Tea & Tango* to Ontario-based Dancing with Parkinson's to branches of Dancing for PD in B.C. and Saskatchewan, are lending a hand in helping Canadians with Parkinson's better manage their symptoms through social dancing.

The colourful background and back stories of Canadian dance studio owners and instructors are outlined. They are as impressive as they are exceptional. If Canada is seen as a country of immigrants, then dance studio owners and their instructors may be seen largely as a tribe of people from the former U.S.S.R., Latin America and western Europe who are totally committed to their art and passionate in sharing their knowledge with social dancers.

A comprehensive list of dance studios in Canada—probably the first in book form—appears at the back. As well, a feature on competitive dancing called "The Thirty-Nine Opinions" is included as an appendix. It is a compendium of varying perspectives by thirty-nine Canadians across the country, about dancesport and salsa competitions which are representations of social dancing.

# Snippets of Our Social Dancing Days and Ways from 1605

# Chapter 1, Part 1: Up to the 17th Century

## Inuit, Métis, And Other First Peoples

The history of *group* dancing and *solo* dancing in Canada goes back thousands of years among Canada's Indigenous peoples.

Through cave drawings of people dancing in a group setting or individually,[1] anthropologists know that humans in simpler societies, like ancient Canada, have danced for a wide range of reasons that include social, ceremonial, and spiritual. They dance to boost fertility; initiate boys and girls into tribal life; select future mates; enter "secret societies;" prepare for war ("war dances"); worship; secure food (hunting, fishing, etc.); exorcise demons; and conduct funeral ceremonies.

Since there have been hundreds of distinct First Peoples in Canada, a correspondingly wide variety of "song and dance" genres exists. This has allowed dancing celebrations and dance forms unique to each and every Indigenous community.

The variations of dancing style have also impacted dancers' regalia. Regalia (clothing, accessories, and artifacts worn or carried) have varied greatly depending on the individuals who have worn it, the culture from which it originated, and the event where it was worn.

The pieces of regalia "tell a story, transmit heritage and serve as badges of honour,[2]" says Amanda Robinson, a researcher for Historica Canada, a nonprofit that researches Canadian history and citizenship issues.

While the energetic and robust dances of Canada's Indigenous peoples[3] are today a delight to behold, it is not entertainment *per se*. It has been an integral part of their lives and is considered by historians and contemporary observers to be inseparable from their music, songs, stories, languages, and culture as a whole.

Here are a few examples of Indigenous nations' dances that exist today but also go back centuries—long before European explorers touched down on the shores of the North American continent.

## Inuvialuit Dancing

The Inuvialuit, a group of Inuit people who live in the Northwest Territories, dance to re-enact their accomplishments from the days of old.

"During celebrations, the blend of the drum beat and the rhythmical rise and fall of voices, punctuated with shouts of *'auu yah iah!,'* quickly [draw] men and women to the dance floor," according to the regional corporation for the Inuvialuit people who live in six communities (Aklavik, Inuvik, Paulatuk, Sachs Harbour, Tuktoyatuk, and Ulukhaktuk, collectively called the Inuvialuit Settlement Region).[4]

Aklavik (population 630), one of the larger communities, hosts the Aklavid Delta Drummers and Dancers. Along with the Ulukhaktuk community, it has been strong in drum dancing.

> This social activity can happen at just about any gathering, including births, weddings, funerals, and to celebrate successful hunts and tourist events. All members of the community can drum dance. Usually Inuit women [sit] in a large circle and [do] most of the singing. The men would drum and dance in the centre.
>
> Dancers would start by offering to do a dance or they could be 'coaxed' into dancing when other men or women would sing a personal song that one of the men had written. The man whose song [is] being sung would then pick up the drum in the centre of the circle and dance and play. Drum dances often [lasts] all night and [include] children.[5]

## Métis Dancing

Another group of Indigenous people, the Métis, have always enjoyed unique cultural traditions. As an Indigenous people of mixed ancestry—Scottish, Celtic, Irish, and French—their dances, especially Métis jigging, are exuberant and link closely with fiddle music.

The Red River jig is the best known and was so named because it originated in the Red River area in central Canada. The jigging dance presents in several forms that include the sash dance, rabbit dance, duck dance, reel of eight, drops of brandy, reel of four, and the broom dance.[6]

For Canada's First Nations as a whole (there are, today, 634 recognized governments)—as well as the Inuit and Métis, a powerful unifying force has been the powwow dances.

Powwows are "musical performances that designate a sense of 'Indianness' based on the common history and dance traditions of Plains[7] culture."[8] Benjamin R. Kracht of Oklahoma's Northeastern State University writes in a journal article.

What takes place in a powwow?

> Dance competitions, special dance demonstrations, initiations, and feasts take place during a powwow ... [Male dances include] Grass Dance, which features movements and regalia that resemble grass swaying in the wind; some believe this dance is done to prepare the grounds for the powwow; Traditional, which evokes a warrior and protector; Fancy, which is energetic and colourful; and Prairie Chicken, which mirrors the mating dance of a prairie chicken. Female categories include ... Traditional, which is grounded in wisdom, grace, dignity, and respect; Fancy Shawl, which personifies beauty and freedom; and Jingle, a healing dance.[9]

According to Canadian powwow observer Paul Gowder, in the twenty-first century there are usually "over 1,000 Native American events listed each year. Every weekend somewhere in the United States or Canada there is a powwow happening."[10]

A good example of dancing at a Canadian powwow is described by Janice Esther Tulk of Memorial University in her doctoral dissertation.

Noting that a traditional powwow is normally held each year in July, Tulk describes what she once saw after the Grand Entry, or opening ceremony, at a traditional powwow of the Miawpukek First Nation reserve on the island of Newfoundland:

> [There was] an intertribal dance open to everyone in attendance, regardless of whether they are wearing regalia. The remainder of the day feature[d] a combination of social dances and category dances. Round Dances, Spot Dances, and Two-Steps [were] interspersed between Men's Traditional, Fancy Shawl, Jingle Dress, and other styles of dance.[11]

The young people at this event were not left out, Tulk says, adding:

While dancers in regalia participate[d] in category dances, participants without regalia dance[d] during social dances and intertribals. Children and youth enjoy a sort of challenge dance that takes place each year, called 'Indian Break dancing,' in which girls face off against boys in a competition to determine who dances the best. Two lines of dancers, one male, one female, face each other.

When the emcee calls forth one female to dance, all of the male dancers must imitate whatever dance move she does. Then a male chooses a slightly more difficult dance step and all the girls must imitate his dancing. This continues as the dance steps become more and more difficult. Audience applause determines the winner and the winning "team" gets bragging rights for the year.[12]

There has been another significant dance common to many First Nations called the round dance. Originally a healing ceremony, the Indigenous "round dance"—for both groups and individuals—has been usually held indoors in the winter.

According to Carleton University ethnomusicologist Anna Hoefnagels, a specialist in First Nations music, singers would strike hand drums in unison and form a large circle with joined hands "symbolically indicating the equality of all people in the circle. The dancers move to their left with a side-shuffle step to reflect the long-short pattern of the drumbeat, bending their knees to emphasize the pattern."[13] It has been a dance for all: children, friends, families, youth, and Elders. Sometimes, non-Indigenous visitors have been allowed to join.

In the twenty-first century, Canadian Indigenous groups and non-Indigenous supporters have also used the round dance to direct their political efforts against provincial and federal governments for land claim rights.

For example, in February 2020, a group of more than one thousand demonstrators carried out a round dance in Toronto in solidarity with the Wet'suwet'en Hereditary chiefs who opposed the Coastal GasLink pipeline company's project that would carry natural gas from Dawson Creek, near the Peace River, to British Columbia's west coast.[14]

The round dance, as a vehicle of protest, helped the nine chiefs, three months later, to achieve a signing of a draft Memorandum of Understanding between the British Columbia provincial government, the Wet'suwet'en Nation, and the federal Liberal government of Justin Trudeau.

The long-standing Indigenous round dance, also referred to in the Plains

Cree dialect as "the tea dance" or "braid bundle dance," is different from the one done in earlier times.

This has come about, according to the Edmonton-based Aboriginal Multi-Media Society, "... after contact with European cultures ... [and as] Aboriginal populations dwindled and eventually became centralized on reserves and settlements, the round dance increased in popularity and size, absorbing many of the ancient dances and rituals" into its current form.[15]

The Indigenous round dance is not to be confused with the conventional non-Indigenous round dance that is popular in square and round dancing circles in Canada (see the social dance chapter in another section of the book.) According to Calgary's non-profit CueSteps Round Dance Club, the round dance "... looks like Social or Ballroom Dancing since the dance rhythms and movements are the same. However, round dancers have the advantage of "pre-choreographed and cued" dances, which use defined (and practiced!) figures/steps...." [16]

# Canada's First Settlers and Dancing in New France

The Mi'kmaq people have lived for hundreds of years in Port-Royal (today, near Annapolis Royal) in Nova Scotia before French explorers established New France, the colony of Canada. As Canada's first newcomers, they established the *first* agricultural settlement in 1605.

Wanting deeply to trade their animal hides and furs with them in exchange for European-made knives and other goods such as iron nails, kettles, and cloth, the Mi'kmaqs forged a working alliance with explorers Pierre Dugua de Monts and Samuel de Champlain.

European-made goods constituted a boon to their lives, and when they traded, their desires were overt and indicated how dancing figured from their point of view: ["In the boats they] showed a marvellously great pleasure in [the] commodities, dancing and going through many ceremonies, and throwing salt water with their hands."[17]

Other French explorers in the sixteenth century who had traded with them and other nearby Indigenous groups such as the Penobscots—earlier called the Etchemins—and the Montagnais (Innu)[18] observed their welcoming attitude expressed similarly: "[They saw] dozens of Indigenous boats coming ... after our longboat, [they were] dancing and showing many signs of joy, and of their desire to be friends."[19]

In his research on dance music in the early centuries of European colonization of Canada, musicologist Helmut Kallmann, a cofounder of the Canadian Music Library Association, discovered similar findings when he learned about French explorer Jacques Cartier's first visit in 1534, noting that "On the arrival of Cartier's ship at the Baie des Chaleurs, groups of Indigenous women and men waded into the sea, jumping, singing, and dancing and making great signs of joy at the visitors' arrival."[20]

Years after 1605, the Mi'kmaqs' lifestyle gradually changed due to the continual French presence and successive waves of new colonists, including the British, Germans, Irish, Scots, Black Loyalists, and Loyalists from the United States.[21]

This Indigenous group has been associated with maintaining stable self-government and loved celebrating life by "holding frequent and lavish ceremonies ... [to pay homage to] "... successful hunts, marriages, funerals, visiting tribes, peace or even war [and featuring] [a] fabulous feast [as] the highlight of these ceremonies, [with] lots of traditional food, song, dance, and laughter."[22]

The Mi'kmaqs had vastly different relationships with European settlers but became increasingly marginalized as the French and British competed with each other for land rights.

European diseases, alcohol, and assimilation strategies, including the arrival of Jesuit priests to convert them to the Catholic faith, inevitably reduced the Mi'kmaqs' capacity to maintain their ways of living, including their ceremonial activities such as dancing.

The conversion of many Mi'kmaqs to Christianity created divisions among them—the converted and the non-converted. For the former, it amounted to "criminalization of Mi'kmaq spirituality."[23]

For the Mi'kmaqs, as a slowly vanishing people due to colonization over the following centuries, it was an important observation about their cultural lives when a priest, Father Pierre Maillard, in a letter to France, noted that an Indigenous shaman once chanted:

> We would dance around the fire, and this is what we would sing: 'Oh Fire, light our pipes and grant that, by sucking in Thy goodness, under cover of the smoke that hides Thee from our eyes, we may become strong and vigorous and always able to know our slave-women and wives of our bed.
>
> May you stay forever in our hearts so that we may never know what is to flinch when we are face to face with those who wish to end our days. Grant that we may laugh and sing and dance when alien executioners wish to dismember us alive.[24]

One of the best overall assessment of the state of dancing in this period for all Indigenous groups at this time is summed up by three writers for the *Canadian Encyclopedia*, who explain:

> Under the impact of centuries of colonization and immigration, Canada's Indigenous peoples retained only a tenuous hold on their once rich dance heritage. Given the often hostile indifference of European settlers to the Aboriginal cultures they disrupted and displaced, and the very different directions in which dance developed in the settler cultures, it was inevitable that Aboriginal dance forms would struggle to have an impact on the later development of dance in French or English Canada.[25]

## The First Social Club Is Set Up

The all-male crews on the ships that brought Pierre Dugua de Monts and Samuel de Champlain to Port-Royal slept in buildings constructed in fortified farm hamlets in Port-Royal, Canada's first agricultural settlement in 1605. So did their leaders, Monts and Champlain. Later, Jean de Biencourt, who succeeded Monts, and Champlain looked to provide a more balanced lifestyle for those under their charge.

Champlain organized a social club called the Order of Good Cheer. The men enjoyed lavish meals through the winter and danced individually to the hurdy-gurdy (a medieval stringed instrument) music while drinking alcohol, which was in great supply.

These events were primarily attended "by the prominent men of the colony and their Mi'kmaq neighbours while the Mi'kmaq women, children, and poorer settlers looked on and were offered scraps [of food]."[26]

In the immediate decades after 1605, many members of the various Indigenous groups living in the vicinity of Port-Royal were influenced by and took up both the music and Catholic religion brought in by the French colonists.

Music generated from the hurdy-gurdy fascinated the Indigenous parents and their children. Sometimes they would ask that "some of our young people should dance to the sound of a hurdy-gurdy, that a little Frenchman held. This was granted them, to their great satisfaction,"[27] a Jesuit priest noted in 1636.

By the mid-eighteenth century, the little settlement of Port-Royal gradually and greatly expanded to encompass a larger Nouvelle-France (New France) territory. The French colonies eventually covered not only the shores of the St Lawrence River, Newfoundland, and Nova Scotia, but also a large swath of the Great Lakes region.

Initially, governing the colonists made up mainly of farmers was King Louis XIV's-nominated intendant, or administrator, Jean Talon. The population was composed initially of small, isolated groups of men travelling throughout the country.

An organized society did not take shape until the creation of the royal colony in 1663, with the establishment of an administration by the Church and the monarchy.[28]

Facing a shortage of women and a desire to rely less on fur-trading and more on agricultural production, Talon actively encouraged the immigration from France of the "King's daughters," a bevy of some eight hundred women, who generally became wives of the male farmers.

## Dancing Was the Colonists' Top Hobby

Although researchers today are now uncovering more details about the dances by the farmers and others in the lower end of society, it is known they certainly did dance "with great vigour and lack of restraint during their several holidays and saints' days in order to forget a while their toil and poverty."[29] Patricia Campbell calls all the dances during Canada's pre-Confederation period "colonial dances."[30]

A major amusement for the nobility—government officials, judges, clergy, and those in the professions—was staging balls. (A ball was defined, in the seventeenth century, as a "social assembly for the purpose of dancing.")[31]

The first ball was held on February 4, 1667, according to Canadian historian Helmut Kallmann,[32] to celebrate the promotion of Louis-Théandre Chartier de Lotbinière to a senior administrative position. The invitees were headed by Daniel de Rémy de Courcelle, the second governor-general of New France, and the rest of the elite members of society.

At this inaugural ball, the partygoers executed several dances, of which the minuet was the most significant and popular. Taking the cue from European countries at the time (where it was the opening dance for all state balls for 150 years from 1650),[33] it started the event.

The minuet's eminence was due to its "balanced, stylized, graceful" look and that it suited the "general spirit of the age" that was characterized by a "certain peace and harmony which went deeper than the mannerisms of the age," British dance historian Frances Rust wrote.

The gavotte, another popular dance at that time, featured sequences such as: "One or two rounds, after which the first leader bows to his lady, performs eight steps in front of her, bows again and then returns to his place with her. All the couples repeat this sequence in succession, then all bow together and take the ladies back to their seats."[34]

They also did other then-popular dances such as the brantle (also called bransle and branle) and courante. In each of these dances, the participants formed a column of couples with the highest-ranking person and his partner in the hall at the head of the line.

During the late seventeenth century to *circa* 1769, Europe saw the adoption of other dance forms and techniques that were partly fuelled by the music within its borders.

For example, the "Folies d'Espagne," a Portuguese dance tune started as a popular dance tune with its improvisational flourishes, transforming existing dances.[35] Early Canadian settlers, whether French, British and others, adapted their dancing to these new techniques. They learned about them from letters and newspapers from their friends and families at their previous European homes.

Among them was the contradanse, also called contredanse, a patterned folk dance from England that was of French origin but had a British beginning (see "Dancing in the Eighteenth century" section later in this chapter).

---

[1] Richard Conniff. "20,000-year-Old cave art from Borneo depicts humans," *Cool Things from the Natural and Human Worlds*. https://strangebehaviors.wordpress.com/2018/11/06/20000-year-old-cave-art-from-borneo-depicts-humans-dancing/

[2] Amanda Robinson. "Indigenous regalia in Canada," *The Canadian Encyclopedia*. https://www.thecanadianencyclopedia.ca/en/article/indigenous-regalia-in-canada accessed 12 June 2020.

[3] In Canada, the term Indigenous peoples (or Aboriginal peoples) refers to First Nations, Métis and Inuit peoples. These are the original inhabitants of the land that is now Canada. In the 2016 census by Statistics Canada, over 1.6 million people in Canada identified as Indigenous, making up 4.9 per cent of the national population. https://www.thecanadianencyclopedia.ca/en/article/aboriginal-people, accessed 24 June 2020.

[4] The Inuvialuit Regional Corporation. https://www.irc.inuvialuit.com/about-irc, accessed 24 June 2020.

[5] *Drum Dance*. http://native-drums.ca/en/music/drum-dance/

[6] The Alberta Teachers' Association. "First Nations, Metis and Inuit Music and Dance", *Stepping Stones*. no. 10, p.3.

[7] The Plains in Canada is a vast northwestern area that includes the Prairies, British Columbia, the Northwest Territories, and Yukon.

[8] Benjamin R. Kracht. "Kiowa Powwows: Tribal Identity Through the Continuity of the Gourd Dance," *Great Plains Research*, vol. 4, no. 2, Aug. 1994, p.258.

39

[9] The Alberta Teachers' Association's *Stepping Stones*, ibid., p.2.

[10] Paul Gowder. Pow Wows.Com. https://www.powwows.com/2020-pow-wow-calendar-experience-native-american-culture-at-an-event-near-you/, accessed 3 July 2020. The Gathering of Nations is the largest pow-wow in the United States and North America. It is held annually on the fourth weekend in April on the Powwow Grounds at Expo NM, in Abuquerque, New Mexico. Over 565 tribes from around the United States and 220 from Canada travel to Albuquerque to participate. Due to the COVID-19 pandemic in 2020, it was cancelled but held virtually and was renamed "Gathering of Nations Virtual Experience."

[11] Janice Esther Tulk. "*Our strength is ourselves: Identity, status, and cultural revitalization among the Mi'kmaq in Newfoundland.* PhD diss., July 2008, p.180.

[12] Ibid., pp.181-182.

[13] Anne Hoefnagels. "Cree Round Dances," *Native Dance*.http://native-dance.ca/en/renewal/cree-round-dances/ accessed 24 June 2020.

[14] Canadian Broadcasting Corporation. "Demonstrators rally, march, dance in Toronto to show support for Wet'suwet'en hereditary chiefs." https://www.cbc.ca/news/canada/toronto/rally-march-dance-wetsuweten-hereditary-chiefs-toronto-support-1.5472838 22 February 2020

[15] Pamela Green and Norman Moyah. "Join the circle—the history and lore of the round dance," *Windspeaker Publication*, vol. 16, no.:2, 1998. https://ammsa.com/publications/windspeaker/join-circle-history-and-lore-round-dance-0, accessed 5 July 2020.

[16] Cuesteps Round Dance Club. https://rounddancecalgary.com/about-us/ accessed 5 July 2020.

[17] Nancy Bonvillain. "The Mi"kmaqs," *Native Nations: Cultures and Histories of Native North America*, Hoboken, NJ: Prentice Hall PTR. p.113.

[18] Daniel J. Weekes. *Gateways to Empire Québec and New Amsterdam to 1664*. Bethlehem, PA: Lehigh University Press, 2019. p.94.

[19] See Ramsay Cook. *The Voyages of Jacques Cartier*. Toronto: University of Toronto Press, p.20.

[20] Helmut Kallmann. "Pre-Confederation Dancing," *The Canadian Encyclopedia*, Pre-Confederation Dancing | The Canadian Encyclopedia accessed 30 June 2020.

[21] Trudy Sable and Julia Sable. "Who we are," *Native Dance*. http://native-dance.ca/en/culturs/mikmaq/who-we-are/ accessed 3 July 2020.

[22] The Confederacy of Mainland Mi'kmaq. *Kekina'muek (Learning)*, October 2007, p.13. https://native-land.ca/wp/wp-content/uploads/2018/06/Mikmaq_Kekinamuek-Manual.pdf, accessed 3 August 2020.

[23] Prosper, Kerry, J. McMillan and A.A. Davis. "Returning to Netukulimk: Mi'kmaq cultural and spiritual connections with resource stewardship and self-governance." *The International Indigenous Policy Journal*, vol, 2, no. 4, 2011, Art. 7, p.7.

[24] This chant is attributed to Arguimaut, a Shaman, and noted by Father Pierre Maillard in a undated letter (but not later than 1758) to Monsieur de Lalane, a senior ecclesiastic in Paris and quoted by Earle Lockerby. "Ancient Mi'kmaq customs: A Shaman's Revelations." *Semantics Scholar*, p.409. https://pdfs.semanticscholar.org/7335/0ed533ae3589b8e40a138a90c160b072d7c1.pdf, accessed 8 July 2020.

[25] Max Wyman, M. Crabb & S.M. Donaldson, "Dance in Canada," *The Canadian Encyclopedia*, https://www.thecanadianencyclopedia.ca/index.php/en/article/dance-history accessed 4 June 2020.

[26] Wikipedia.
[27] Father La Jeune, report 14 August 1636, *The Jesuit Relations*, vol. 9, p.269.
[28] Library and Archives Canada. "Daily life" Daily Life - Library and Archives Canada (bac-lac.gc.ca), accessed 5 September 2020.
[29] A.H. Franks. *Social Dance: A Short History*. London: Routledge & Kegan Paul, 1963, p.26.
[30] Patricia Campbell, "18th Century or Colonial Dances." https://countrydancecaller.com/18th-century-or-colonial-dances/, accessed 23 September 2020.
[31] Nathan Bailey, *An Universal Etymological English Dictionary*, 1742.
[32] Helmut Kallmann, op.cit.
[33] Frances Rust, *Dance in Society: An analysis of the relationship between the social dance and society in England from the Middle Ages to the Present Day*, p. 60.
[34] A.H. Franks, ibid., p.77.
[35] DanceTime Publications. https://dancetimepublications.com/resources/social-dance-timeline/late-17th-century-18th-century-circa-1685-1769, accessed 29 June 2020.

# Chapter 1, Part 2: The 18th and 19th Centuries

## 18th Century Canada: People, Economy, and Social Dancing

About one quarter of the population of New France lived in towns where people were royal officials, military officers, merchants, or artisans. As in the latter part of the previous century, most people were farmers growing wheat, peas, oats, rye, barley, and maize on long, narrow farms huddled along the St. Lawrence River.

"Some of the biggest entrepreneurs in Québec City and Montréal were women. Marie-Anne Barbel, for instance, presided over a fur trading business, a pottery works, and large real estate holdings."[1]

The latter part of this century saw shifts in dancing forms following the Seven Years' War that ended in 1763. The British defeat of the French in that war was confirmed with the Treaty of Paris. All of French North America east of the Mississippi River was ceded to Britain, with the exception of the tiny islands of St. Pierre and Miquelon off Newfoundland.[2]

A net result was an exodus of French people; of the 30,000 French who made the voyage to New France between 1604 and 1760, roughly half chose to remain.[3] At the same time, there were increased flows of English and European immigrants into Canada.

## The Most Popular Ballroom Dances

The new wave of immigrants from England brought the "ballroom [country]" dances most popular there and in Europe at the time. The first half of the eighteenth century was dominated by the Morris dance,[4] bourrée, passepied, and the rigaudon (also called the rigadoon).

The Morris dance involved rhythmic steps with the dancers usually wearing bell pads on their shins.[5] Implements such as sticks, swords, and handkerchiefs were sometimes carried by the dancers. A French folk dance, the bourrée was characteristically danced with quick, skipping steps.[6]

With the dancers dressed as shepherds and shepherdesses, the passepied featured the feet crossed and recrossed while gliding forward, one foot often striking the other. It evolved, liked the minuet, as a couple dance with figures.[7] The rigaudon was a sprightly seventeenth century French folk dance for couples. Its hopping steps were adopted by the skillful dancers of the French and English courts.[8] During the course of the century, the contredanse, cotillion, and allemande became popular.[9]

The British country dance genre, a characteristic form of folk and courtly dances,[10] took a strong hold in France (also in Portugal and Denmark) after the 1690s as contredanse anglaise and were renamed contredanse française and later called simply contredanse. It is to be noted the British country dances were a simpler version in step patterns of Irish set dances and Scottish country dances.[11]

The French cotillion, a specific contredanse—with a "square for 8" dancers—was greeted with great enthusiasm by the English.[12] As well, the allemande, earlier adapted by France from Germany, was an "export" by French dancers to their English counterparts.[13] This dance featured the chassée, a basic step involving a changing step to the side, now a staple move in today's international slow waltz and cha-cha.)

New musical expressions also developed, as in the decades before, transforming dancing forms and techniques. "[A] particular feature of dancing in the eighteenth century was this individual creation of dances to fit one particular type of music," dance historian Frances Rust notes. Using the bourée as an example, she says it could not be danced to the music of another. "Sometimes a dance would take on a multiple form, a combination of several dances in one, for example, sarabande-bourée."[14]

During this century, says square dance historian Dorothy Dahm of Tillsonburg, Ontario, Canada and America also saw the beginnings of square dancing.[15] She cites the cotillion and "longways—dances done in lines with partners facing each other—as the "grandfather" of today's square dances.

The French colonists' passion for dance in early Canada was easily matched in the last decade of the century by the English. The wife of John Graves Simcoe, Upper Canada's (Ontario's) first lieutenant governor, continued the tradition of staging balls following their arrival from England in 1792. Multitalented Ms. Elizabeth Posthuma Simcoe—a prolific diarist and watercolourist—took every opportunity to organize balls and attend dance events she did not organize.

Evidence of this Upper Canada's First Lady's indulgence in dancing can be seen in her entries for a ten-day period in 1792, the first year of her stay in Canada.[16]

On January 21, 1792 she wrote:

> Miss Johnson dined with me & we went to a dance in the Evening at the Fusileers' Mess Room—very agreeable.

On January 24, 1792:

> I gave a dance & supper to a dozen of the Fusileers & as many young dancing Ladies. My Rooms being small obliged me to invite so few & only those who dances.

On January 31, 1792:

> A very pleasant dance at the Château this Evening

Two weeks later, in a letter to Mrs. Hunt at Wolford, England, Simcoe wrote, "I never was so free from colds as I have been this winter tho' I dance a great deal & leave hot rooms without wrapping myself up, as is the way here."

# 19th Century Canada: People, Economy, And Social Dancing

Pre-Confederation English Canada, after the British took over the territories previously run by the French in 1760, was marked by a gradual shift in the economy.

The Industrial Revolution was well underway. Steam power enabled machines to produce goods much faster and less expensively. Thus, the economic landscape focused more on manufacturing and services than on agriculture and extracting resources such as gold, silver, zinc, iron, copper, and nickel.

An increasing number of people earned their living by working for someone else, although many others were independent farmers, fishermen, and craftsmen. But those who were employees, the so-called working class, were in the majority. They emerged as a result of "the spread of industrial capitalism in British North America."[17]

Until the 1780s, there was no significant European population in Upper Canada (present-day Ontario). However, the population spiked with the steady arrival of United Empire Loyalists (UEL) refugees (American residents of all races and economic classes who were loyal to British rule), British and American settlers, and British troops and officials[18] who opposed the American Revolution.

By 1821, York (now Toronto) had grown to over 1,500 residents. According to Toronto historian Edith G. Firth, Toronto evolved from being a "small, undistinguished village" in 1815 to become a "booming city" in 1834.[19] Immigration had multiplied its population thirteenfold and had greatly altered the background and outlook of its residents.[20]

In contrast to the 1830s, the population of Toronto at the beginning of the second decade consisted of a "small, self-conscious upper class composed of senior government officials and military officers, with a larger group of 'shirt-tail' relatives and hangers-on connected with it.

"The majority of residents, however, were working men, small shopkeepers, artisans, and minor civil servants, many of them discharged soldiers," writes Firth.

There was no substantial middle class, she adds. "Immigration made few additions to the upper class, which had become a closed circle, solidified, ingrown, unsusceptible to outside influence."[21]

The economy of Québec (after the 1760 British takeover of New France from the French administrators), which was largely based on military spending and the fur trade, changed too. Mining copper, gold, zinc, forestry, dairy farming, and fishing became increasingly important as British Canadian and American investors learned.

In Western Canada (Manitoba, Saskatchewan, Alberta, and British Columbia), settled agriculture began in 1812 at the Red River Colony.[22] This development can be viewed as a copycat version of the first agricultural settlement in Port Royal in 1605 during the time of the first French colonists. The building of the Canadian Pacific Railway in the 1880s boosted the Prairies' wheat economy.

(Earlier in the west, economic development began with the fur trade. By the end of the eighteenth century, Métis and First Nations peoples on the prairies engaged in the trade. Fur-trade posts were scattered throughout the region; on Vancouver Island, the city of Victoria began as a Hudson's Bay

Company trading post.)[23]

In the Atlantic provinces, after the British defeated the French, the colonies remained mostly vacant until the aftermath of the American Revolution (1775–83) but saw a large influx of United Empire Loyalists' migrants from the United States. They developed this region into "a thriving community of English loggers, fishermen, and shipbuilders."[24]

## Technology Spreads the Popularity of Dancing

Recreational pursuits across the country were, generally, the same. Rail travel, starting in the 1880s, increased the speed with which new dances spread.[25]

Juliet McMains, a dance professor at the University of Washington who has competed in Canadian DanceSport competitions, explains how technology quickly disseminated dancing knowledge across the North American continent:

> The new recording industry offered much cheaper alternatives to live music, increasing the number of people who had access to dance music.... Not only was the music itself the vehicle through which dances migrated, but dance instructions also found new homes on record jackets and even oral instructions on the records themselves.[26]

In rural areas, according to historians, the life of pioneer settlers was one of hardship, but "the difficulties under which they lived were to some extent relieved by cooperation, not only in work but in play."[27] ("Bees," for example, where people gathered and worked together for a communal purpose, were common.)

Although most ordinary people in nineteenth-century Canada carried out their daily lives almost the same as those decades earlier, they engaged in several harmful habits. Among them were abuse of alcohol at weddings, auction sales, and other social gatherings, smoking, robberies, profanities, lawlessness, wrestling, and fighting. In Upper Canada (Ontario), these occurrences were plentiful.[28]

Despite that, dancing was of paramount importance in their social life.

The aristocratic manners that included bows and curtsies in a dance ball were practised by elite members of society. Especially from the beginning of the reign of Queen Victoria of England in 1837 until 1901, fashionable social dancing in Canada was "courtly."

Although not "elite" in the sense that it enjoyed the wealth, prestige, and leisure time associated with the privileged few, a growing middle class in cities took up those Victorian rules of dancing. The motive was for people to make themselves more acceptable in places such as Toronto, Hamilton, Montréal, and Vancouver.

Early in the century, elegant dances such as the waltz were done mainly among the upper-class members of society. However, in Canada, with an expanding middle class, the waltz became—as in Europe after the French Revolution in the late 1790s—a popular democratic dance that allowed social dancers outside elite circles to participate.

Those who lived in rural areas, representing the vast majority of the people, mainly danced the country dances (as defined by the English and later by the French).

"Of all the amusements of early times, dancing was the most universal and appears to have given the greatest pleasure to the greatest number," says Canadian historian and educator Edwin C. Guillet.

They executed their versions of English country dances, focusing on square dancing. However, observers noted they danced in their own way; "more exercise than grace" was the order of the day.[29] Among the dances were the Scotch and Irish reels, four-hand and eight-hand reels, jigs, and hornpipes.[30]

For both elite members of society and the upwardly mobile who lived in the towns, dancing schools set up shop to support the learning and practice of the waltz, the minuet, and quadrilles.

For example, in York (Toronto), between 1825 and 1925, there were no fewer than thirty dancing schools, according to York University dance professor Mary Jane Warner.[31] There was also the itinerant dance instructor group who could not obtain permanent employment and travelled to towns where there were few dance schools. Some of these teachers, called "dance-masters," placed advertisements "in the local newspapers giving the beginning date, location and place to obtain admission tickets for classes."[32]

A typical advertisement for dance students in Toronto read like this:

> Mrs Charles Hill's
> Academy for Dancing & Calisthenics
> Is Open for Adults from Eight to Ten
> every Monday and Wednesday.
> Juvenile Class, from Three to Five
> every Wednesday & Saturday.
> Schools and Private Families attended.

> Mrs Charles Hill attends a Class
> every Tuesday and Thursday, at 3 o'clock at the
> Academy of Madame Delande, by whose kind permission
> Pupils in the vicinity of York Street may Attend
> Toronto, 18th Dec., 1849[33]

Another advertisement, from 1845:

> Mr. A.C. Fitch
>
> Begs to inform the Ladies and Gentlemen of Toronto
> that he has, since the 18th instant,
> opened a Dancing School. At the large Ball Room of the
> North American Hotel, Front Street.
> Mr. F. will teach the Polka, Polka Quadrilles, Mazourkas, &c.
> For Terms, see Cards. Residence at McDonald's Hotel
> Toronto, August 21, 1845[34]

In Hamilton, Ontario, members of the upper class did not have to travel fifty-eight kilometres to Toronto for dance lessons and entertainment. Freda Crisp in Toronto discovered in 1991 in her research that from 1840 to 1860 the popularity of social and theatrical dancing as entertainment for Hamilton's elite grew primarily from "from the need and desire for recreational activity." She notes in her university thesis:

> Social dancing lessons as part of polite learning were vital to the cultural development of Hamilton's upper class. Through the study of ballroom dancing (which took place under a dancing master), the City's upper class attained cultural refinement, which was a necessary requisite to membership in polite society. Dance was emphasized in the pursuit of social graces because it was in the ballroom that the upper class was on its best behaviour.[35]

Perhaps prototypical of the dancing life of some upper-class citizens in Canada is the social activities of a twelve-year old boy who arrived in Toronto from England in 1833. Larratt William Violet Smith, who eventually became vice-chancellor of the University of Toronto, was an inveterate partygoer.

His diaries are a testament to his life as a socialite, with many entries relating to dancing, dance types such as quadrilles, bands, music, and, more importantly, attendance at parties.

Smith's entry on February 21, 1840:

> Raining almost all day yesterday. Went to the office till ½ past 1—came home and rode out on Tomi's poney to Mr. Boyd's party at Richmond Hill. Rain in the evening prevented many coming, but the Duries, the Gappers, the Barwicks, John Pareson, Mrs. and Miss Cameron all came.[36]

A diary entry for November 1840 reads:

> Thursday 26th. Very fine & colder. Went to Stanton's party last evening, very crowded but very pleasant. The 34th Band played quadrilles for the first time… [W]ent to Mrs. Robinson's in the evening. The 32nd band was there with violins, etc. Introduced to Miss Foster by John Robinson, & to Miss Turquand by Miss Robinson. I also danced with Miss Heath and the third Robinson daughter. Came home at ½ past 2 after a very pleasant evening indeed.[37]

Another entry from December 28, 1843:

> Snowing, sleeting & raining all day. Went to the office as usual. In the evening I took Mary & Miss Thomson to a party at Mrs. Cozens. Wore my white neckcloth in public for the first time. It was a splendid evening. I danced with a good many ladies & had great fun with Miss Thom.[38]

## Following the Rules of the Dancing Game

Like the highly organized social dance "balls" common to the upper strata of society, starting with the ones in seventeenth-century New France, the elites in both Québec and Upper Canada (Ontario) continued the tradition their predecessors followed: staging lavish balls in "assembly rooms" that contained a ballroom and even a tea room and lounges, and in the drawing rooms of private homes or clubs such as curling, cricket, golf, and sailing.

According to a present-day U.S. ballroom dance competitor who has done extensive research on that era, a standard program for a mid-nineteenth-century ball consisted of a mazurka, polka, waltz, and cotillion.

Julie Malnig, writing in *Dancing Till Dawn*, outlines the sequencing for dancers: "This sequence of dances was usually decided in advance by the hostess and listed on dancing cards given to all the guests. The steps of the dances were performed in a fixed order … [with] out-turned feet and pointed toes. The physical stance of the social dancers themselves was prescribed and proper."[39]

For the elites during this period, the cotillion, a group dance involving regular interchanges of those on the dance floor, was the most popular. The cotillion was usually placed last in the dance sequence. Along with parlour games, this dance provided opportunities for socializing among couples.

For those who were single, dancing brought together people "of similar backgrounds, often for purposes of introducing young men and women of marriageable age."[40] Coming-out balls, debutante balls, or cotillion balls were standard events by the mid-1800s.[41]

Such social activities, however, did not have free run. Like the rest of the world, Canada was experiencing the continual effects of the Industrial Revolution, political changes in England, and the increasing power of the Church.

During the reign of Queen Victoria of England (1837–1901), for instance, the Methodist churches and the Church of England in Canada were front-and-centre in instituting higher standards of moral behaviour. As an example, "...legions of guides were published on how to behave correctly, how to dress appropriately and what to say in various specific situations."[42]

Dancing and etiquette manuals set precise standards in the way men and women should interact on the dance floor and the ceremonial details for conducting oneself for ballroom. These included the etiquette of how to invite guests to a ball, requesting a partner to dance, and no-nos while conversing on the dance floor.

William Warwick, a nineteenth-century Toronto publisher who distributed the *Canadian Ten Cent Ball-Room Companion and Guide to Dancing*, joined in the fray. He outlined, among other things, rules of dancing etiquette and ideas for running private parties.

His suggestion on how "gentlemen" should dress:

> He should wear a black dress-coat, black trousers, and a black or white vest, as suits the taste of the wearer; a white necktie, white kid gloves and patent-leather shoes.
>
> This, in the 'best society,' is imperative. The ball-suit should be of the best cloth, new and glossy, and of the latest style as to cut. The vest may be cut open or low, so as to disclose an ample shirt-front, fine and delicately plaited; it is better not embroidered, but small gold studs may be used with effect.[43]

Warwick's prescription for ladies' "toilettes," meaning "the whole complex of operations of hairdressing and body care that centered at a dressing table,'"[44] stated:

> A lady, in dressing for a ball or party, has first to consider the delicate question of age; and next, that of her position, whether married or single.
>
> As everything about a ball-room should be light, gay, and the reverse of depressing, it is permitted to elderly ladies, who do not dance, to assume a lighter and more effective style of dress than would be proper at the dinner-table, concert, opera.
>
> The toilette of the married and unmarried lady, however youthful the former, should be distinctly marked. Silk dresses are, as a rule, objectionable for those who dance; but the married lady may appear in a moire [silk with a rippled look] of a light tint, or even in a white silk, if properly trimmed with tulle and flowers.
>
> Younger unmarried ladies should wear dresses of light materials—the lighter the better. Tarlatane, gauze, tulle, aerophane, net, the finest muslin, lace and all similar fabrics...[45]

Maud C. Cooke, an American journalist and an authority on etiquette, agreed with Warwick in the way women should dress for balls. She pointed out in her book on "polite society" published in London, Ontario, in 1896, that sophistication is a key element:

> For the ball-room the most elaborate dress is to be worn; décolletté [low neckline] corsage, flowers, and jewels are all appropriate. Those who dance should wear pale colors and light, floating fabrics, leaving the heavy silks and velvets for those who do not indulge in this amusement.
>
> A low-cut corsage is not expected of elderly women unless they wish it. Chaperons can wear an elegant dinner dress if they desire; velvets or brocades, cut square in the neck, with profusion of fine lace and rich ornament....
>
> If an elderly woman of full figure wears a low-necked dress, a lace scarf or something of that sort should be thrown over her shoulders.
>
> Gowns cut dancing length or with a train, are appropriate for the ball-room, but where much dancing is to be indulged in, trains are very much in the way.[46]

## The State and Churches: Opposition to Dancing

In 1831, Canada's population had just passed one million, and at the time of Confederation, it rose to 3.4 million.[47] The country also saw the first signs of a growing population mosaic that consisted primarily of English, French (particularly in Lower Canada [present-day Québec]) and German residents.

The changing in composition of the peoples' country of origin inevitably led to some tensions between their religions and perspectives on life, including social dancing.

However, dancing has long been a sticking point in many societies. It has been vilified since the fourth century, and according to specialist dance researcher Mark Knowles, who writes on the history of negative reaction to the waltz and "scandalous dances," anti-dance sentiment reveals "the shifting social ideologies of the day."[48]

Canada's Indigenous groups did not escape the wrath of social changes. In 1884, the federal government outlawed the "potlatch" ceremony usually celebrated by Indigenous peoples. This move was part of its policy of assimilating First Nations groups into Canadian society. The ceremony involves spirit dances, feasting, gift-giving, and community building activities. "The government and its supporters saw the ceremony as anti-Christian, reckless and wasteful of personal property," says René R. Gadacz. "They failed to understand the potlatch's symbolic importance as well as its communal economic exchange value."[49]

For sixty-seven years following the introduction of the potlatch legislation, many criminal charges were instituted against First Nations by the Canadian authorities. Among the arrested were forty-five Kwakwaka'wakw (Kwakiutl) in 1922. Defending themselves, the Kwakwaka'wakw "insisted that in their religion '[a] strict law bids us dance,' but to no avail."[50]

By the late 1830s, Upper Canada had a diverse religious scene. The Church of England, Quakers, Mennonites, Irvingites, Campbellites, Mormons, Methodists, and others dotted the landscape, providing what Canadian historian Gerald M. Craig calls "the gospel to a pioneer community, as well as a stimulating social occasion to lonely men and women from the backwoods and an excellent opportunity for courtship for young people."[51]

The Methodist churches were particularly vocal about what they called the evils of dancing. Said Reverend Richard Hobbs, in a Sunday sermon on March 1, 1896, to his congregation in Brantford, Ontario:

> I declare to you that such amusement as the pleasure of dance of today is a curse to the race, a libel on Christianity, and a

dishonor to God.

> It is argued that our young people must have recreation, and therefore the dance is the best way to recreate themselves.… I assert, then, if they take the exercise that the dance demands of them, they are sinning against their physical, intellectual, and moral well-being.[52]

Fifteen years earlier, a contemporary colleague, Reverend W.J. Hunter, offered another argument against dancing as a justification for acquiring what he called "elegance of manners." Preaching at his church on Bloor Street near present-day Bay Street, the minister clarified his point:

> I am not prepared to deny that the art of dance, as now taught, embraces many good lessons in politeness, and that it does impart a certain ease and gracefulness of manner; but it is not necessary to go to a dancing-school, or to attend dancing-parties, in order to acquire ease and gracefulness in society. There are thousands of ladies and gentlemen who have never danced, and whose elegance of manners no one will question.[53]

Referring to the First Ladies of American presidents, the minister said:

> Those amiable and accomplished ladies, Mrs. President Hayes and Mrs. ex-President Polk, of the United States, while receiving and treating guests with great kindness and politeness, have never permitted dancing in the White House during the terms in which they have presided over its social ceremonies.[54]

H.T. Crossley, a leading Methodist evangelist during the last quarter of the century, visited every Canadian city, except Québec City, during his mission for Christ, offered a messaging strategy that dancing is "paltry, frivolous, illogical, and unchristian."[55]

Crossley's *Eleven Rejoinders* [author's emphasis] to eleven "excuses" he had heard from dancers during his travels were summarized in one of his writings, *A Practical Discussion of the Parlor Dance, the Theatre and the Cards* (that is, card playing):

> *First excuse*: "People must have amusement and recreation." Certainly, but look at the dancers next morning, you will conclude that dancing is not recreation, but dissipation.
>
> *Second excuse*: "People might better dance than do worse. They might better dance than slander others or have kissing plays." Yes, but if you stop dancing, you do not have to do worse. Can

you not keep slandering your neighbour in some other way? Kissing plays among adults are a thing of the past, or are only found among the most illiterate and uncultured.

*Third excuse*: "Dancing is an accomplishment." ... Nay, it prevents many from seeing how little mind they have, and the necessity of acquiring true accomplishment... Dancing is a sort of subterfuge for those who lack mind.

*Fourth excuse*: "If I don't dance, I cannot pass in society." ... The best society does not dance instead of demeaning yourself by running after a certain "upper ten" society ... showing yourself to be of such intellectual, social, and moral worth, that even the so-called "upper ten: will rise in their ideal of life, and aspire to pass in your society.

*Fifth excuse*: "All my associates, and the people I visit, dance." Then, let me assure you have a grand opportunity, instead of being led by others, to show your independence of mind and strength of character....

*Sixth excuse:* "When I hear music my feet begin to move." ... Let your feet move ... that is natural; but that has nothing to do with encircling a lady's waist with your arm, or having a gentleman's arm encircling your waist.

*Seventh excuse*: "I dance, and my conscience does not condemn me." So much the worse for you, when the spirit of Christ and His Word show that you are wrong.

*Eight excuse:* "If we do not dance or play cards, what shall we do when spending an evening?" ... [G]et more brains. A vacant mind leads to the ruin of many. Those who have the fewest brains are most enamored with the "light fantastic."

*Ninth excuse*: "Our church and clergymen are not opposed to dancing." The particular congregation where you attend church, and your misinformed, worldly, or patronizing clergyman may disagree your Church and its ministry by sanctioning the dance; but let me ask you to follow the teaching and example of the many great and good, who are worthy representatives of your Church, who are most pronounced against the dance.

*Tenth excuse*: Some say "The modern dance has the sanction of Scripture." ... Did you notice that this religious dancing [referred to in the Scriptures] is altogether unlike our modern dances. It was (1) outdoors; (2) in the daytime; (3) spontaneous; not prescribed; (4) skipping or tripping, as children, expressive of religious joy; (5) women and men separate, and not men and women in each others' arms, as in the modern dances. (6) the religious dance of the Bible was a natural expression of religious joy and praise to God, to celebrate the victories of the Lord and of Israel—the modern dance is but a means of personal carnal amusement and worldly pleasure; (7) the religious dance of the Bible is no more our modern dance, than the sacrament in church is like a drunk carousal in a bar-room.

*Eleventh excuse*: If the Church opposes dancing, the young people and others will be kept from being members… It is evident that the churches that are most opposed to the dance … have the largest number so youth and adults join their membership.[56]

## Prince Charles Dancing with the Locals: The 1860 Royal Tour

According to the *Canadian Encyclopedia*, the British monarchy has been arranging tours to Canada (then British North America) since the late eighteenth century. The earlier tours were political as they "focused on the relationship between the monarchy and the military, while later tours included diplomacy, philanthropy, and the Crown's relationship with Indigenous peoples."[57]

In 1860, Albert Edward, the Prince of Wales, the eldest son of Great Britain's Queen Victoria, arrived in Canada on the first official Royal Tour of Canada. Describing the young prince as one of the world's wealthiest men at the time "with a playboy reputation and zeal for dancing," *Toronto Sun* journalist James Wallace, in a historical piece for his paper, wrote in 2017 that when in Toronto, the young prince indulged in dancing, one of his favourite hobbies, at Osgoode Hall (a two-and-a-half-storey building in downtown Toronto built in 1832) on September 8, 1860: "[T]he Prince, as he had elsewhere on his Canadian tour, indulged his fondness for dancing which he did until close to midnight. At a subsequent ball, he danced until 4:00 a.m."[58]

Another ball, the Citizen's ball in Toronto, held on September 11, 1860, was held at the Royal Canadian Yacht Club in his honour. A special notice was issued by the "military secretary" located at 149 College Street in Toronto, advising "ladies attending the dance" that they would have to embark at the Harbour Commissioners' Wharf at the foot of Bay Street at 8:45 p.m., and dancing was scheduled for two hours—from 9:30 p.m. to 11:30 p.m.

The young prince's passion for dancing with locals at a grand ball when he first arrived in Canada at St. John's was reported in North American newspapers. Taking a cue from this, more than two dozen mayors across Ontario (then Canada West), in preplanning for the eventual arrival of the prince, placed public balls as one of the top welcoming events.

According to University of Toronto historian Ian Radford, who spent years researching and writing about the prince's activities in Canada during the summer and fall of 1860, notes how the ball organizers made special arrangements for both married women—in the main—and young women to be the Prince's dance partners.[59]

(Prince Charles also attended, during this tour, grand balls organized by Newfoundland and the maritime colonies of Nova Scotia, New Brunswick, and Prince Edward Island.)

## Dining, Drinking, and Dancing Close to Confederation (1867)

The now-famous Fathers of Confederation who negotiated the process that eventually led to the creation of the Dominion of Canada on July 1, 1867 were thirty-six colonial politicians representing the existing British North American colonies at the time.

Between 1864 and 1866, the politicians held meetings and "conferences" starting in Charlottetown, Halifax, Saint John, Fredericton, Québec City, and ending in London, England. The London Conference eventually led to the proclamation by the British Parliament of the *British North America Act* creating Canada.

While the politicians intensely debated the issues around a possible Confederation, they also found time for socializing between meetings and travelling by steamship, rail, and horse-drawn carriages between the cities. In fact, Canadian historian P.B. Waite, known for his analyses of the events leading to Confederation, has argued that "[I[t would be fair to say that the delegates spent nearly as much time, if not more, dining, drinking, and dancing, than they did negotiating, at least officially. And oh, the parties were spectacular."[60]

On October 14, 1864, a grand ball held in Québec City for the delegates of the Québec Conference catered to eight hundred people. According to research reported by *Canadian Stamp News*:

On the evening of the 14th a very brilliant Ball was given in the Parliament Buildings, under the auspices of the Canadian Ministry," said Prince Edward Island delegate Edward Whelan, who was also a journalist and advocate for responsible government. "It was attended by the same classes—the same distinguished persons and society as attended the 'Drawing Room' on the 11th.

His Excellency the Governor General [Lord Monck], His Excellency the Lieut. Governor of Nova Scotia and Lady, the Members of the Canadian Government, the Delegates from the Eastern Provinces, and about 800 others, formed a large and most agreeable party, by whom the pleasures of the dance were kept up without interruption and without an incident to mar the harmony of the occasion, until nearly 3 o'clock on the morning of the 15th.[61]

Another grand ball with dinner and dancing was held weeks before at the Colonial Building in Charlottetown, Prince Edward Island, during the Charlottetown Conference held September 1–9.

This meeting, known officially as the Charlottetown Conference, was called by politicians from the colony of Canada (now Québec and Ontario) to discuss a "union" of the Maritime colonies (excluding Newfoundland at the time).

According to the diary of Mercy Anne Coles, the daughter of George Coles, a PEI delegate: "On Tuesday, September 6, Edward Palmer (a PEI politician) gave [a] luncheon and the lieutenant-governor and his wife gave a grand ball at Government House in the evening."[62]

Although there is no official record of the proceedings of this conference, research has recently come to light indicating that dancing and socializing were forefront activities at the gatherings of delegates.

"The Islanders, it turned out, including the PEI politicians, were more interested in the circus [that had arrived in town] than in the negotiations to unite the colonies," claims Anne McDonald, a Saskatchewan award-winning author and theatre instructor, whose book *Miss Confederation: The Diary of Mercy Anne Coles*[63] analyzes the behind-the-scenes activities of the twenty-three delegates.

"You can't blame them," McDonald suggests. "The late summer was as lovely as summer can be in what's come to be known as Canada's Garden Province, and the circus was the highlight of the season."

## Dancing After Confederation (1867)

The creation of the Dominion of Canada on July 1, 1867 saw a union of New Brunswick, Nova Scotia, and the Province of Canada (Québec and Ontario). Joining the Dominion later were Manitoba and Northwest Territories, which eventually split into the present-day territories of Yukon and Nunavut, and the provinces of Alberta and Saskatchewan. British Columbia, Prince Edward Island, and Newfoundland were the last provinces to join the federation.

The provinces and territories' desire to be one nation reduced the possibility of being assimilated by the United States.

Capitalizing on the fervour for nationhood, Canadian governors-generals engaged the power of dancing and social entertainment as a political tool. Lord Aberdeen, who was governor-general from 1893 to 1898, and his politically active wife Ishbel Maria (she organized the National Council of Women in Canada and other major national associations) realized that fancy dress balls were a powerful way "to feed Canada's growing nationalism" and to shape Canada's identity.[64]

Lavish entertaining with fancy dress balls—and there were four of them between 1876 and 1898—as the innermost element were the order of the day. Naturally, journalists had a field day with these events, since the general population was eager to know about the "symbolic costumes, historical themes, the commemorative album, and even the use of a triumphal chariot [that] evoked the spirits of pageantry and Renaissance spectacle."[65]

The vice-regal entertainments—and there were others but less elaborate—also affected the local economy of the three hosting cities. Analyzing the Toronto Victorian Era Ball, held in 1897 to celebrate Queen Victoria's Diamond Jubilee, researcher Janet Wason notes that beyond the effects of learning about the historic, symbolic or fanciful costumes worn by attendees, "[T]his elite entertainment affected the lives of many of Toronto's population, for the newspapers were unanimous in their praise for the monetary benefit it brought to the trade and service sectors."[66]

Although the invitation lists to major social gatherings at Rideau Hall (the official residence of the governor-general in Ottawa) were generally limited to the *crème de la crème* of society (such as cabinet ministers, senators, members of Parliament, high-level civil servants, judges, doctors, and lawyers), the governors-general did allow the general citizenry to sign the guest book at Rideau Hall in the hope of securing an invitation to major entertainment events. Among them were shopkeepers, butchers, bakers and grocers.[67]

[1] Library and Archives Canada. "Daily life in New France," http://www.canadahistoryproject.ca/1663/1663-14-daily-life.html, accessed 20 September 2020.
[2] Brittanica, *"Royal Control",:* https://www.britannica.com/place/Canada/Royal-control, accessed 23 September 2020.
[3] Library and Archives Canada, "Survival," https://www.bac-lac.gc.ca/eng/discover/exploration-settlement/new-france-new-horizons/Pages/survival.aspx, accessed 22 November 2020.
[4] "A folk dance." Ibid.
[5] Anonymous. *Open Morris: A short history of morris dancing,* https://open-morris.org/morris-dancing/, accessed 2 September 2020.
[6] Editors of Encyclopaedia Brittanica, "Bourree," https://www.britannica.com/art/country-dance, accessed 3 September 2020.
[7] "Passepied dance.", https://www.britannica.com/art/passepied, accessed 3 September 2020.
[8] "Rigaudon dance." https://www.britannica.com/art/rigaudon, accessed 3 September 2020.
[9] Rust, op.cit. p.59.
[10] Editors of Encyclopaedia Brittanica, "Country dance: British dance." https://www.britannica.com/art/country-dance accessed 3 September 2020.
[11] op.cit.
[12] Rust, op.cit., p.61.
[13] Ibid., p.62.
[14] Ibid.
[15] Dorothy Dahm. htpps://swosda.ca/history. accessed 1 September 2020
[16] Mary Quayle Innis, ed. *Mrs. Simcoe's diary.* Toronto: Macmillan of Canada, 1965.
[17] Dimitry Anastakis, "Industrialization in Canada," *The Canadian Encyclopedia,* https://www.thecanadianencyclopedia.ca/en/article/industrialization, accessed June 3, 2020.
[18] Ian M. Drummond & Ford Macintosh, "Economic history of Central Canada," *The Canadian Encyclopedia,* https://www.thecanadianencyclopedia.ca/en/article/economic-history-of-central-canada accessed June 27 2020
[19] Edith G. Firth, "The Town of York `1815-1834," The Champlain Society for the Government of Ontario. *The town of York 1815-1834: A further collection of documents of early Toronto.* University of Toronto Press, 1966, front flap
[20] Ibid., p.lxxx
[21] Ibid., p.lxxxiii.
[22] Ian M. Drummond & Ford Macintosh, "Economic History of Western Canada," *The Canadian Encyclopedia,* https://www.thecanadianencyclopedia.ca/en/article/economic-history-of-western-canada accessed 20 June 2020.
[23] Ibid.
[24] Anon. "Atlantic Canada," The Canada Guide. https://thecanadaguide.com/places/atlantic-canada/, accessed 11 October 2020
[25] Juliet McMains. *Glamour Addiction: Inside the American ballroom dance industry,* Middletwon, CT, Wesleyan University Press, 2006, p.68.
[26] Ibid.
[27] Edwin C. Guillet, *Early life in Upper Canada.* Toronto: The Ontario Publishing Co. Ltd., 1933. p.295

[28] Ibid., pp.298-300.
[29] Ibid., p.310.
[30] Guillet's research reveals great details of a typical dance meet. He writes: "Above the noise of the dancing could be heard the scraping sound of the fiddle, and the voice of the caller-off as he shouted "Salute your Partners," "Promenade All," or "Grand Chain." Some rustic dancers called for equally rustic directions from the caller-off, whose shouts, "Balance to the next and swing out", "Gents hook up, ladies bounce back," "Down the centre and chaw hay," usually exhibited more ingenuity than gentility. Among the popular dance music of pioneer days were prominent *The Soldiers' Joy, Money Musk, Old Dan Tucker* and *Pop Goes the Weasel*.
[31] Mary Jane Warner, *Toronto Dance Teachers: 1925-1925*, Arts Inter-Media Canada/Dance Collection Danse Press/es. Toronto, 1995, pp. 85-92.
[32] Ibid. p.11
[33] *The Globe*. 20 November 1849, p.92.
[34] Advertisement. *British Colonist*, 21 October 1845.
[35] Freda Crisp, *Dance in polite society* Hamilton, Canada West, 1840-1860. MFA thesis. Toronto: York University, 1991. https://elibrary.ru/item.asp?id=5824816, accessed 2 July 2020.
[36] Mary Larratt Smith. *Young Mr. Smith in Upper Canada*. Toronto: University of Toronto Press, 1980, p.35.
[37] Ibid., p.47.
[38] Ibid., p.93.
[39] Julie Malnig, *Dancing Till Dawn: A century of exhibition ballroom dance*. New York, New York University Press, 1992, pp.2-3.
[40] Anon. "Ball Dress," *Encyclopedia of Clothing and Fashion*, vol.1. New York: Charles Scribner's Sons, 2005, p.112.
[41] Ibid., p.112.
[42] Karine Rousseau, "Balls (In the 19th and early 20th centuries)." Montréal: McCord Museum. http://collections.musee-accord.qc.ca/scripts/explore.php?Lang=1&tablename=theme&tableid=11&elementid=83__true&contentlong, accessed 20 September 2020.
[43] WM Warwick. *Canadian ten cent ball-room companion and guide to dancing, comprising rules of etiquette, hints on private parties, toilettes for the ball-room, etc. Also a synopsis of round and square dances: diction of French terms, etc.* Toronto: WM Warwick, 1871, p.9.
[44] Anonymous. "Jane Austen's world," https://janeaustensworld.wordpress.com/2011/09/30/an-18th-century-ladys-toilette-hours-of-leisurely-dressing-and-private-affairs/, accessed 24 July 2020.
[45] WM Warwick, ibid., p.8.
[46] Maud C. Cooke, "Social etiquette, or, manners and customs of polite society: Containing rules of etiquette for all occasions," London, ON.: McDermid & Logan, 1896, p.416.
[47] Warren E. Kalbach, "Population of Canada," *The Canadian Encyclopedia*. https://www.thecanadianencyclopedia.ca/en/article/population, accessed 2 November 2020.
[48] Mark Knowles, *The wicked waltz and other scandalous dances: Outrage at couple dancing in the 19th and early 20th centuries*. Jefferson, NC: McFarland & Company, Inc. 2009, p.1.
[49] René R. Gadacz, "Potlatch," *The Canadian Encyclopedia Note:* The ban on the potlatch was lifted in 1951.

https://www.thecanadianencyclopedia.ca/en/article/potlatch, accessed 3 November 2020.
50 Jordan D. Paper. *Native North American religious traditions: dancing for life*. Westport, CT: 2007 p.xii.
51 Gerald M. Craig. *Upper Canada: the formative years 1784-1841*. Toronto: McClelland and Stewart. 1963. pp. 166-169.
52 Rev. Richard Hobbs, *The evils of the modern pleasure dance: A sermon preached by the Rev. Richard Hobbs: Colborne Street Methodist Church, Brantford*: Strathroy, Ont.? s.n. 1904?
53 Rev, W.J. Hunter, "The pleasure dance in its relation to religion and morality: *A sermon preached in Bloor St. Methodist Church, Yorkville on Sabbath evening, Jan. 30th, 1881.*" Toronto: Methodist Book and Pub. House, 1881. p.11.
54 Ibid.
55 H.T. Crossley. *A practical discussion of the parlor dance, the theatre, the cards*. Toronto: William Briggs, 1895, p.15.
56 Ibid., pp 8-15.
57 Carolyn Harris, "Royal tours of Canada" *The Canadian Encyclopedia*, https://www.thecanadianencyclopedia.ca/en/article/royal-tours, accessed 20 July 2020.
58 James Wallace, "Prince Albert was first British royal to visit Canada in 1860," *Toronto Sun*. 2 July 2017
59 Ian Radford, *Royal spectacle: the 1860 visit of the Prince of Wales to Canada and the United States* Toronto: University of Toronto Press, 2004. p.151.
60 P.B. Waite. *The life and times of Confederation 1864-1867: Politics, newspapers and the union of British North America*, Montréal: Robin Brass Studio, 3rd. ed., 2010.
61 Canadian Stamp News. https://canadianstampnews.com/grand-ball-hosted-for-delegates-of-quebec-conference-1864/, accessed 5 January 2021.
62 Anne McDonald. *Miss Confederation: The diary of Mercy Anne Coles*. Toronto: Dundurn, 2017, p.39.
63 Ibid.
64 Cynthia Cooper. *Magnificent entertainments: fancy dress balls of Canada's Governors General 1876-1898*. Fredericton, N.B.: Goose Lane Editions; Hull, P.Q.: Canada Museum of Civilization, 1997.
65 Janet Wason. "The Victorian era ball," in Selma L. Odom & Mary J. Warner. *Canadian dance: visions and stories*. Toronto: Dance Collection Danse, 2004, p.71.
66 Ibid.
67 Cynthia Cooper, op.cit., p.xvii.

# Chapter 1, Part 3: 20th Century to the Present

## 20th Century Canada: People, Economy and Social Dancing Life

As the twentieth century dawned, Wilfrid Laurier, Canada's prime minister from 1896 to 1911, governed a vastly transformed modern country.
- Fifty per cent of Canadians lived in urban cities and towns by 1910 (Newfoundland and Labrador, and Nunavut joined Canada in 1949 and 1999 respectively);
- Between 1901 and 1911, there was population growth of nearly 3 per cent each year through immigration—mainly to the Western provinces. By the end of the First World War in 1918, the population was 7.2 million;[1]
- Factory industries arose in every corner of the country and for those served by long distance all-year round railway routes and good roads, the country's economy grew leaps and bounds;
- (It was only in the Great Depression years—the 1930s—and during the difficult years between the First and Second World Wars, according to historian Paul-André Linteau, that Québec "reached its first significant watershed on the long road to modernity.");[2] and

- Big banks and investment houses, focusing on metropolitan areas such as Toronto, strengthened the country's financial base.

The social landscape also saw dizzying transformations due to larger trends: the women's rights movement took off, rallying for social and sexual freedom; middle- and upper-middle classes of people increased in numbers; and a consumer culture became firmly established with the growth of the advertising industry.

The demand for leisure and entertainment opportunities grew alongside these developments. Swept along the currents of change, the social dance scene became altered forever. The changes amounted to a "social-dance revolution."[3]

In the twentieth century, "ballroom" as a term loosely applied to all social dances, began a period of unparalleled rapid development. The growth manifested itself in several ways:

- Dances initially adopted by the Canadian upper class since the seventeenth century became popular with middle classes and eventually cascaded down to ordinary Canadians.
- A virtual torrent of new dances started in the "ragtime" era, leading to tango and later to salsa—the focal points of this book. In the meantime, square dancing continued as it had been since 1605 (when Canada's first permanent agricultural settlement was established).

# From the 1900s until the Second World War

The passing of Queen Victoria of England in 1901 released social dancers from the strict Victorian rules and moral codes for those in the fashionable ballroom. Writes Theresa Jill Buckland, a dance professor at England's Roehampton University, of that time "The ballroom of the upper and middle classes increasingly became a space for young men and women to express themselves more freely in movement."[4] The latter began "doing their own thing" in the sense that they made changes "not only in the order direction of steps, but in the style and variation of the steps themselves."[5]

That, they maintained, was the more modern and natural way to dance. Expression of individuality was rife, to be in vogue with the ideals of the Progressive Era (the social activism and reform period in the United States from 1890s to the 1920s) that spread to Canada and the United States.

Dance scholar Juliet McMains sums up the turnaround in the M.O. (*modus operandi*) of dancing:

> Nineteenth-century social dances required that all members of the group perform their part in the predetermined sequence of steps and trajectory through space. In contrast, the new twentieth century ballroom dances gave little prescription for a single couple's relationship to the rest of the group.[6]

In England, United States, and Canada, younger dancers rejected the sequenced group round dances (quadrilles, waltzes, lancers, and the like) of earlier generations in favour of being able to navigate alone as couples on the dance floor. Thus, improvisation (doing a dance figure without preparation) and playfulness became the norm.

At the same time, musical developments such as Afro-American ragtime music—most popular between 1895 and 1919 in the U.S.— were embraced by Canadians. For example, a handful of Canadian composers such as R. Nathaniel Dett and Willie Eckstein[7] reacted dutifully and created classic rags so people could dance to the new musical fad. Ragtime music in Canada fed social dancers' desire to self-express on the dance floor, as well as inspired a menagerie of "animal dances" such as the grizzly bear, turkey trot, and bunny hug throughout North America.

Across Canada, adolescents ten to nineteen years of age were spending much of their leisure time apart from their families. Many enjoyed the myriad new dances coming on stream. They danced during all types of events, including dinners. "[T]here were certain dances that caught on [among] the younger generation … [but] some of these dances were considered scandalous and inappropriate," writes Ellen Arual on her "Canada's Entertainment in the 1920s" website.[8]

Arual did not clarify what her descriptors "scandalous" and "inappropriate" meant. Observers have speculated that people, particularly those in the upper and upper-middle classes, did not approve of their daughters or wives engaging in the animal dances. These new dances, at that time, were considered licentious because they involved extremely close dance holds and positions.

A spokesperson for a major American dance association reportedly said, "The turkey trot was "absolutely vulgar … The dancing is from the hips up, instead of from the hips down, as is proper … It is not so much what the Turkey Trotters do with their feet. That does not count. It's the position which lends to vulgarity."[9]

One researcher put it more bluntly: these dances were filled with "a lot of hugging, swaying and grinding to the strong rhythms of the music."[10]

One of the results of the runaway nature of dancing during this period was the emergence of the concept of "modern" ballroom dancing. English dance teachers became scared they would be out of work unless they tamed the beast of improvised dancing. In response, their professional associations pushed to standardize the dances: this meant steps, techniques, and conventions had to be set out and reinforced by a syllabus, examination standards, and licensing of teachers.

Reforming the dances, which had implications for social dancers in the United States and Canada, according to a University of Washington's dance professor, also implied a colonial mindset and racial considerations. Juliet McMains explains:

The need to prescribe behavior for colonized peoples in everyday life was reflected in the efforts to redefine these newly colonized dances. Movement of nonwhite bodies and nonwhite movement practices had to be carefully ordered by British rule in order to ensure continued domination and submission.[11]

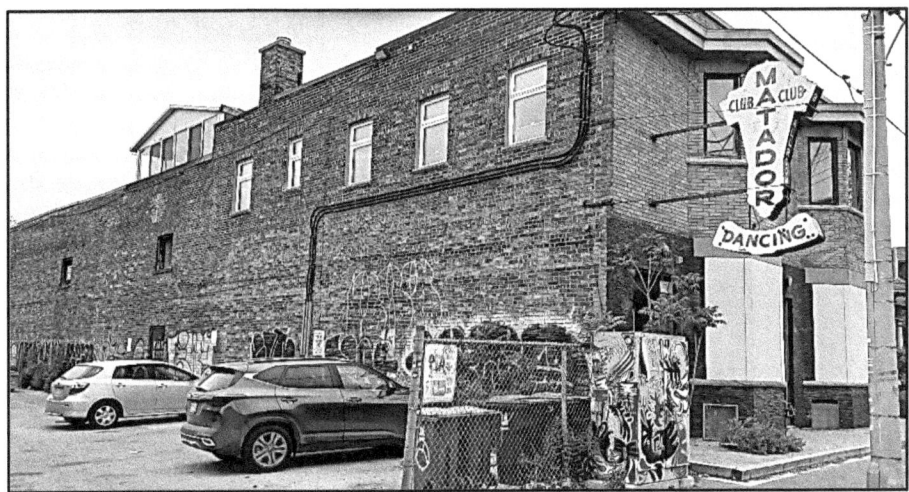

Figure 1: The shuttered 105-year-old Matador building, a historic landmark, at 466 Dovercourt Court in Toronto was initially the Davis Assembly Hall and served as a community dance hall during the First World War. The first owner of the building was dance teacher Charles Freeman Davis, the eldest son of John Freeman Davis, the patriarch of a family of ballroom teachers.

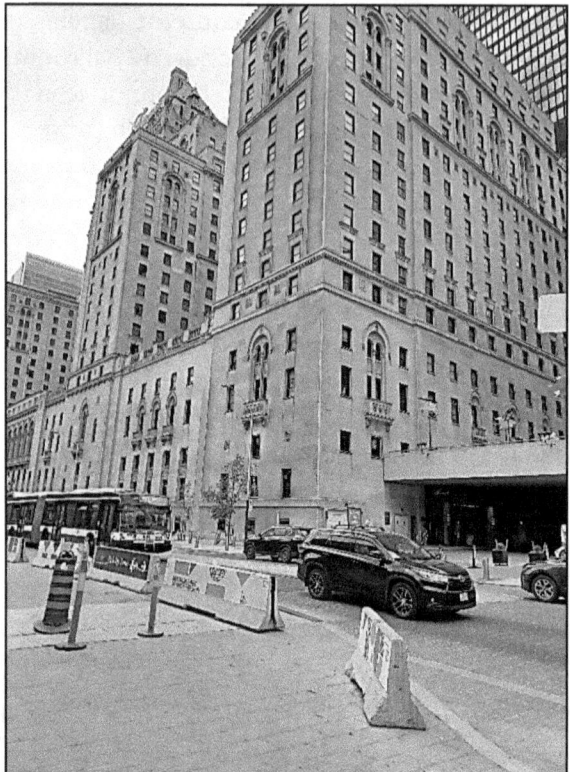

Figure 2: The imposing 28-storey Fairmont Royal Hotel, commonly known as the Royal Hotel, is located at the southern end of Toronto's financial district. In the 1930s the hotel's ballrooms were well known for grand balls attended by Ontario's dignitaries, celebrities.

## Latin Dances Appear

While the upper- and upper-middle-class members of Canadian society ambled on with the fashionable round dances (the quadrilles, waltz, lancers, and similar dances) of yesteryear, a flurry of dances coming out of the Afro-Caribbean and Latin America appeared in Paris and London, as well as in North American cities.

Among them was the ballroom tango, which was imported to America from Buenos Aires via Paris by several dance instructors, among whom was an American married couple, Vernon and Irene Castle. After learning the tango and other new dances in Rochester and other U.S. cities, itinerant dance instructors in turn travelled to Canada to teach their enthusiastic dance customers.

The tango was "the first Latin dance to make a significant and lasting appearance in European and American ballroom," says dance scholar Juliet McMains. "The year 1913 is often singled out as the height of this tango mania."

The "wicked" tango, as was stereotyped by the media, first caught on in Québec. And it created quite a stir.

According to P. O'D, a dance columnist for Toronto's *Saturday Night* magazine, the largest city in Canada was "pure and unspotted" until Montréal took to the tango lock, stock and barrel. In a 1913 critique, he wrote tongue-in-cheek:

> Well, when Montréal started to indulge in pastimes so immoral—anything that interferes with digestion as these restaurant dances must, is bound to be immoral—we knew that Toronto would not long resist. And after all the easiest and safest way to resist temptation is to succumb to it. So, Toronto succumbed.[12]

"Tangomania" swept swiftly across Canada from Newfoundland and Labrador to British Columbia. The young and the old of all social classes could not resist its power. Quite democratizing a dance it was!

One young lady in Newfoundland, self-identifying as "Distressed," seemingly was not lucky to get her mother to allow her to attend tango parties. In a letter to advice columnist Annie Laurie in St. John's *The Daily Mail* in 1914, she wrote:

> My mother says that anyone who dances the tango ought to be ashamed. She lets me waltz and two-step all right but she's been somewhere and heard some creature talk about the tango so she thinks it's awfully wicked.
>
> Nobody does anything but the tango and I am absolutely for it, for mamma won't let me go anywhere where they tango.[13]

As for the other Latin dances such as the rumba and cha-cha, this period also saw plenty of fans drawn to them. These dances resonated with people because "they capitalized on their reference to non-Western, non-white culture."[14]

In high-society public entertainments such as "state balls,"[15] the tango was shut off in 1914. Learning about "tangomania's" popularity in Canada, the Duchess of Connaught, the vice-regal consort (the wife of Governor-General Prince Arthur, First Duke of Connaught and Strathearn) banned the dance forthwith. Reporting on the development, a dispatch from a correspondent for *The Globe* read in part:

> The tango, mild or otherwise, will not be tolerated at Rideau Hall [the official residence of the Governor-General]. Not that there has been any definite instructions that the latest craze is unacceptable to their Royal Highnesses, but it has been quietly but effectively made known to those members of society who have the honor of being invited to the dinner dances at Government House that the Duchess of Connaught disapproves of any of the many tango steps being introduced in the ballroom.[16]

A group of Ottawa women who had formed a tango club were obviously disappointed. The duchess's decision also hit them hard in the pocketbook; they had pooled money to hire a tango consultant from New York to teach them the 120 tango steps. Classes had already started when they heard the tango was banished from Government House.[17]

At the turn of the second decade of the twentieth century, the so-called "Roaring Twenties" (or the "Jazz Age") began. It was a period of economic prosperity following the First World War in 1918, and ended with the 1929 Wall Street Crash (the American stock market disaster that saw stockholders losing their shirts).

Canadians who once embraced the "animal dances" earlier later took to jazz music and the new dance moves associated with it, such as the Charleston (featuring fast leg swings, big arm movements, and hand clapping), and the black bottom (based on the Charleston).

While jazz and the new dancing it spawned took the U.S. by storm, Canadians also took to them. According to Carissa Wong on her website,

> Jazz, as a revolutionary form of music, became extremely popular in Canada. Blending European and West African music styles, its strong and rhythmic beat continued to emerge in popular music today. Jazz artists like Louis Armstrong, Bessie Smith, and Duke Ellington became famous and, with the help of radio, helped the Jazz Age to spill over into Canada.[18]

After picking up the steps for the Charleston and black bottom in the growing number of dance schools, especially in fast-growing Toronto, people from all social classes practised the moves both at home and in public dances.

## Montréal Develops a Reputation for Jazz Nights

Quoting an Afro-American historian, tap dancer and Afro-American dance researcher Cheryl M Lewis described jazz as having "developed a reputation for good times in an era when Prohibition was inhibiting night life everywhere on the continent."[19]

> In 1922, there were twenty-three commercial broadcasting stations in Canada. By the late 1920s, radio sets using loudspeakers were widely available, attracting middle-class persons who could afford them, restaurants, clubs, and taverns, which wanted to attract customers, and remote towns and localities.[20]

While Canadian radio stations expanded their reach and helped arouse people's interest in dancing, films, and Hollywood musicals featuring dance, such as *Dance Hall* (1929) and *The Spanish Dancer* (1923), had a similar impact. (The first public screening of a film in Canada took place in Montréal on June 28, 1896.)[21] During the 1920s, Canada had around 451 theatres across the country, and they featured the dozens of 1920s movies coming out of Hollywood.[22]

With Prohibition (the government ban on the production, importation, transportation, and sale of alcoholic beverages in the U.S.), Montréal became internationally known as a go-to haven for tourists seeking relief from "the strictures of temperance."[23]

But Canada did not escape the temperance movement against alcohol; there were, in fact, local government bans in the late nineteenth century, as well as provincial bans in the early twentieth century. Besides, Canadian prohibition was short-lived—only from 1918–20—except Prince Edward Island, which repealed it twenty-eight years later.

During Prohibition, secret clubs, called "speakeasies," sprang up all over Canada. Club meetings were held at the back of stores or even underground and featured drinking bootlegged liquor, gambling, and dancing.[24]

Outside of the period of Prohibition, social dancing was one of the few legitimated means to enjoy nighttime recreation.

If it were thought that men generally did not like to dance, the Charleston was the one dance that saw a breakthrough for men, says Mark Knowles of U.S. males, "College boys, athletes, policemen, waiters, princes—all wanted to learn the snappy dance."[25] Canadian dancers followed suit.

The waltz and tango continued, with slow waltz becoming a new trend. The foxtrot became smoother than the earlier short-stepped version. Other ballroom dance forms prevalent during this period were the one-step and the maxixe (Brazilian tango). The Brazilian samba was introduced in Paris in 1922 and then spread to North America.[26]

## Ballroom Dances and the Dance Industry in the 1920s

Expanding cities and towns across Canada led to increased opportunities for dance teachers and studios. Social dancing became a viable industry and more mature—with an increasing number of dance teachers, dance schools, public dance halls, dance literature, dance performers doing cabaret shows, seamstresses making dance dresses, and cobblers adjusting shoes for dancing.

In her 1990s research on Toronto's dancing scene during this period, York University dance professor Mary Jane Warner identified dozens of Toronto ballroom dance teachers such as Charles Freeman Davis, H.H. Corfan, Jean Whyte, Charles J. Viola, W.J. Sheppard and many others[27] who formed the core of the ballroom dancing academy.

They promoted the standards[28] established in England during the 1920s by the top dancing associations led by the Imperial Society of Teachers of Dancing.

People of all social classes in Canada danced together in public dance halls. And dance school advertising promoted the idea that dancing was an elixir: it would imbue one with class, grace, and a romantic halo. In other words, dancing was viewed by many as a gateway to higher social status and personal popularity.

The larger cities were dance-crazy after hours on weekends. In Toronto, many working-class people could not have enough. Daytime dancing started. The *Toronto World* newspaper reported, "We hear of the 'tango' this and the [waltz] 'hesitation' that. And now we have added a few dancing hours to the day by having dancing luncheons."[29]

In search of constant self-improvement, large numbers of people who could afford dance lessons enrolled. Progressive-minded women who sought personal freedom from the years earlier found dancing more liberating than before: they dressed in shorter skirts to reveal their ankles and trimmed their hair short, and they went dancing unescorted.

Never in the history of dress has the dance played so important a part in the making of modes.

It has compelled changes from the most unexpected sources and has stamped its influence on the dress of young and old.[30]

## 1940s to 1960s: Good Dancing Times for Urban Masses

The Great Depression (or "Dirty Thirties") caused prices and profits to plummet in every area of the Canadian economy. Being dependent on farm and resource exports to Britain and the U.S., whose economies had been devastated, Canada experienced massive unemployment. What was even worse was the so-called Dust Bowl, a series of dust storms that severely damaged major crops in the Prairies.

Labour statistics showed almost one-third of the labour force was out of work and one-fifth of the population had to rely on social assistance.[31]

Millions of people—mainly women and girls—were forced to stay at home. The more resilient ones found ways to combat potential mental health issues by turning to recreation and leisure pursuits at home and church functions.

For working young women at that time, the Depression limited their free time and available money. However, they also made time to have fun, consort with boys, and still be respectable and safe in urban centres, according to Katrina Srigley, a professor at Ontario's Nipissing University in her study of the 1930s. "In domestic spaces young women listened and danced to music played on the piano, gramophone, and radio."[32]

At other times, when girls did in fact go out in groups and encountered boys, as they did a lot in Ontario through the Toronto Rough 'n' Ready Spinsters' Club, they socialized.

At dances everywhere in the province, they danced endlessly. But the young women who preferred the ballroom dances might have found the boys wanting in ballroom skills—at least in the London, Ontario, area. In the 1930s, the conservative local board of education passed a resolution to disallow its young women teachers from teaching "older boy students the art of ballroom dancing."

As one of his legacies, C.C. Carrothers, outgoing board chairman, pronounced that ballroom dancing "certainly can't help discipline", and so quashed a motion commending teachers for their dancing instruction.[33]

Hotels were quick to spot opportunities to profit from the public interest in dancing and the expanding music scene punctuated by travelling dance bands that were popular through their radio work, music recordings, and live appearances. The pumped-up big beat of the music on weekends was irresistible. Quoting a young Toronto woman for her research, Srigley learned that dancing "bedazzled the single working woman."[34]

The largest hotels in Canada made special arrangements to host regular visits of orchestras. This in turn was a magnet for dancers from all around. In Toronto, the Royal York Hotel (now the Fairmont Royal York Hotel) and the King Edward Hotel; in Montreal, the Windsor Hotel and Mount Royal Hotel; the Château Frontenac in Québec City; the Nova Scotian Hotel in Halifax; the Empress Hotel in Victoria, B.C., and Hotel Vancouver, also in B.C.[35]—and their large ballrooms overflowed with guests. These events, patronized to the hilt by upper and upper-middle class people, such as well-to-do brokers, professionals, real estate dealers, and factory owners, enabled them to mix readily and have fun.

In Toronto, Canada's largest city, the Palace Pier and Casa Loma offered an equivalent classy ambience to the hotels and so attracted a high level of clientele.

Although Toronto's Palais Royale was generally cheaper to get in and was a favourite among all classes of people, the dance hall management in the "Palais" and some other dance halls denied entrance to Black couples.

> While no ethnic enclave had a monopoly on dancing, couples were denied access to dance halls in Toronto because of their racial identity.
>
> For instance, black Torontonians were not welcome at the Palais Royale. When Count Basie, a popular black American big-band player, was performing at the dance hall in 1939, the youth of the Toronto United Negro Improvement Association (UNIA) decided to picket the establishment. They did not have success....[36]

New dance halls were built and existing buildings converted to dance halls. Outside the perimeters of larger cities, wooden summer dance pavilions went up in large numbers, dotting the Canadian landscape from Vancouver to Toronto.

Author and communications consultant Peter Young has identified two dance pavilions and dance halls in Ontario that drew Ontarians in droves for social dancing between 1930 and 1960. As he rightly notes in the preface to *Let's Dance,* he "recalls the places in which we [Ontarians] loved to swing and sway, as well as the legendary entertainers [orchestras and singers] who made us dance."[37]

There were so many of them he organized them geographically with descriptions in a dozen chapters:

- Toronto and surrounding areas (16 pavilions and dance halls)
- Around the Bay by Burlington to the shores of Lake Erie (15)

- Across Southwestern Ontario from Woodstock to Amherstburg (16)
- Owen Sound to the shores of Lake Huron (14)
- Brantford north to the Georgian Bay area (32)
- Around Lake Simcoe (11)
- Through the Haliburton Highlands into the Kawarthas (7)
- Peterborough and surrounding areas (14)
- The Ottawa Valley to the Seaway Valley (27)
- Central Lake Ontario area (28)
- Muskoka area (1) and
- Near North (10).

For teenagers and young adults, the pavilions became not only a venue for dancing but also a new place to look for relationships. Young Baptists found them to be an "ideal location for respectable courtship."[38]

In the western provinces, social dancing also thrived.

"Every Friday and Saturday night during the 1930s and 1940s in southern Alberta everybody danced … or so the story goes." With that line, University of Lethbridge theatre professor Lisa Doolittle reveals in her study that social dancing in western Canada was a parallel phenomenon to Ontario during most of the same period.

According to Doolittle, the Trianon Ballroom dance hall in Lethbridge, Alberta's third largest city, opened in 1931. This dance venue eventually paved the way for the opening of hundreds of little Trianon-like dance halls across Canadian prairie towns during the following two decades.[39]

(The "Trianon Ballroom" is the generic term to describe many dance halls that cropped up during the Big Band era of music in the United States and Canada.)

Citing small southern Albertan towns and hamlets near Lethbridge such as Burdett, Champion, Enchant, Maple Grove, Willow Creek, and Whitla that held community hall and outdoor pavilion dancing events, she calculated there was a dance hall for every four thousand inhabitants in towns and an even higher proportion in the rural areas.

The Trianon Ballroom in Vancouver opened two evenings before the 1918 New Year's Eve celebrations. The *Vancouver Sun*'s headline read: "Magnificent New Ballroom Open Tonight" with a picture describing the dance floor: "Six thousand feet of dance floor of the latest ship-deck spring type await the eager feet of Vancouver dance lovers."[40]

Vancouver's Alexandra Ballroom was the venue of the historic first appearance of one of Canada's leading dance bands, Mart Kenney and His Western Gentlemen, in 1931. Soon Kenney was touring around B.C. and Alberta, pulling in the masses with a sweet sound popular with dancers.[41]

Another historic first appearance of a top big band in Alberta, with a huge crowd of dancers, to raise money for a local Board of Trade's community efforts took place in Bassano, a town southeast of Calgary, on Friday, April 12, 1940. The Sunny Fry Orchestra then left for engagements in eastern Canada at various lakeside resorts.[42]

The Trianon Ballroom in Regina opened its doors in December 1929: The first dance was sponsored by the Alexandra Club with the Dave Mills Orchestra. Some of the liveliest dances, according to one observer, were held when soldiers returned home after 1945. According to Joy-Ann Cohen, a columnist for the *Leader-Post*, during the Depression years and after the Second World War:

> There were many single persons around who didn't know anyone, [during the Depression years and after the Second World War], and they came to the Trianon to make friends.
>
> Before the [Second World] war, 'stag' girls never came; after they would enter in groups of four or five, and the returned soldiers flocked to the hall to meet them...
>
> In the early days, Tuesday nights were reserved for whist [card games] and round dances, Thursday nights for whist and old-time dances (square dances, polka) and Saturday nights for round dances only.[43]

Public interest in dancing in commercial dance halls was particularly heightened when U.S. dance bands visited major Canadian cities. The Duke Ellington Orchestra, for example, appeared in Toronto on May 25, 1954, then three days later at the Sherbrooke Arena in Québec on May 28. Travelling westward, the band played at the Calgary Stampede corral on June 20, following by an appearance at Regina's Trianon Ballroom on June 29.[44]

Service-oriented community groups also held regular dances in regular "non-Trianon" pavilion settings. One of the thousands of such events was hosted by the Rebekah Lodge in Lethbridge. At the K. of P. hall, the dance was reported to be "delightful" and attended by one hundred and fifty couples. It took place two weeks after New Year's Day in 1918.[45]

In cities such as Edmonton, there was growth in the number of dance schools to meet the high demand for group classes. Dancers' enthusiasm even extended to learning exotic dances such as the Russian Walk. This advertisement[46] appeared in a *The Wetaskiwin Times* in Wetaskiwin, a city of south of Edmonton, on January 19, 1922:

> Mrs. and Miss Lotta Boucher School of Dancing, Edmonton.
> Mr. H. Boucher will commence in the Angus Hall
> Wednesday 25 January
> Class work, including Waltz, Waltz Hesitation, Rye Waltz, Fox Trots (3), One Step (2), Two Step and Three Step.
> Terms—6 class lessons $10.00
> (We guarantee to teach you in in the 6-lesson course)
> Private Tuition —$2.00 one half hour
> Folk dancing and National Dances for children and young people will be taught if a class can be formed.
> Can you dance the "Russian Walk" as danced in New York?
> We teach it—$5.00 per couple

In French Canada, Catholicism had a strong grip on the everyday existence of its adherents during the first third of the twentieth century. Catholics lived a traditional way of life based on the social values of the Church.[47] This region of Canada was thus not part of the widespread and large-scale appearance of public "social dancing" in English-speaking Canada.

On the other hand, there was plenty of public socializing. Like elsewhere in Canada, they certainly headed to the taverns. Québec, which adopted prohibition in 1919, quickly repealed it after the public put pressure on politicians to do so. As a result, the province became "known as the "sinkhole" of North America [and] [t]ourists flocked to "historic old Québec.""[48]

In the eastern provinces, Nova Scotia's Cape Breton step dancing—a traditional dance form emphasizing footwork brought in by Scottish immigrants decades earlier—was prevalent. The quadrilles and lancers forms of dancing were imported in the 1920s but were molded to "their manner of dancing … [by] marking "rhythm of the music with the toe and heel beats and brushing movements" instead of walking through the quadrille and lancer sets, as was done elsewhere.[49]

The places where this Cape Breton version of the new dances also changed.

Before the turn of the twentieth century, most dances were held at home gatherings or during weddings. Gradually, dances were held in schoolhouses (normally to raise money to maintain the school), in parishes, and community and private halls. The first of these public halls was likely built in the 1930s or 1940s.[50]

## Drinking and Dancing

Along with the growth of public dance halls—which normally involved the sale and drinking of liquor during events—provincial governments created regulatory agencies for the sale and consumption of alcohol.

In 1927, the Ontario government created the Liquor Control Board of Ontario (LCBO). According to Brock University professor Dan Malleck, the LCBO sought to:

> ... separate the consumption of alcohol from other forms of leisure pursuit. Notably, it tried to eliminate the association between drinking and other stars in the constellation of vices [drinking, smoking, taking drugs, ambling, sexual misbehavior, and swearing—vices attributed to American author John C. Burnham in his book, *Bad Habits*].[51]

As it worked toward facilitating public drinking in licensed beverage places, the board faced a major challenge: how to prevent people from going to illegal venues that encouraged singing, dancing, and playing games while drinking.

It also had to contend with hotel owners who were not happy campers because they were not denied licences allowing drinking and dancing in their dining rooms.

The hotels near the Detroit River argued that sizeable revenues from drinks and entertainment sales were being lost to roadhouses on the U.S. side of the international border; visiting American businessmen were known to have booked guest rooms for the night all right but spent their evenings drinking and dancing at the roadhouse bars.

During the debates on the issue, the government received torrents of complaints from the Arlington Hotel, Bridge Ave. Inn, British American Hotel, and St. Clair Hotel in Windsor; Riverside's Edgewater Hotel; Ottawa's LaSalle Hotel; St. Catharines' Ontario Hotel; and Niagara Falls' Royal Hotel.

The owner of the St Clair Hotel once told an LCBO inspector about the unfairness of having U.S. roadhouses compete with them, and groaned, "[I]f it were not for the dancing I am afraid I would lose all my business as I would be the only hotel on River Road that did not have music and dancing."[52]

# From 1960s to 2020s: Growing and Maturing

During this sixty-year period, there was tremendous flux in the social dancing scene.

In addition to the many new social dances such as the shim sham shimmy line dance (1930s), the jitterbug, a swing dance variant (1930s–40s), the hand jive—usually danced to rhythm and blues music, the twist, a favourite among teens (before Chubby Checker popularized it in the 1950s[53], and rock 'n' roll—there was a wellspring for even more in the following decades.

In the 1960s, for instance, the swim, pony, frug, mashed potato, shake, chicken and dog dances and twist dances became well liked, fueled by a strong interest in funk and soul music.

The 1970s saw disco music spawning dances such the hustle, the "YMCA," the funky chicken dance, and the bump.[54]

During the following two decades, the cabbage patch, running man, roger rabbit, snake, and moonwalk dances (popularized by pop star Michael Jackson) attracted many social dancers.

## Public Funding for Training Young Bodies and Minds for Dancing

Support for pre-university dance education has been fragmented across the country. Many training and education school boards have placed dance in the arts area, where it competed with better known and established forms such as music, painting, and photography, while others have located it within physical education, including sports.

In deciding which arts activity got appropriate attention and funding, school officials have often left out dance.

As with other dance genres, ballroom dance was not officially included in school until the late 1990s and still does not have a teaching syllabus for the educational system in this country, says former York University graduate student David Outevsky, who in 2018 obtained his doctorate writing about Canadian dancesport.[55]

The overall result of the hit-and-miss attention to dance funding in the elementary and secondary school systems has generally resulted in only small numbers of Grade 12 graduates, until the late 2010s, having knowledge or skills in social dance as they leave school to begin working or starting up their college or university education.

Since 2007, Ilsa Abraham, a Toronto-based job development specialist, and school vice-principal Robert Rutherford followed on the footsteps of Pierre Dulaine, the 1994 founder of Dancing Classrooms in New York, by launching a similar project in Ontario to encourage school children to dance socially.

Abraham's nonprofit corporation cooperated with the Toronto District School Board, Canada's largest (almost 600 schools), to have six schools take part in ballroom and Latin dancing lessons for Grade 5 and 6 students.

Karen Albertson, a former vice-principal of École Winchester Public School in Toronto, described her school's participation in the dance project:

> Dancing Classrooms is one of those opportunities that create a supportive and positive environment to nurture respect and civility amongst the students, while meeting the Ontario curriculum expectations across all areas.
>
> It is also excellent professional development for the classroom teacher to work alongside professional dance artists. Parents are equally enthusiastic about the program. It brings meaningful connections between home and school when the students practise the dance steps at home with their parents, or when we host ballroom dancing family night.[56]

As if underscoring the buzz that was created by Abraham's project, hailed as "an innovative character development program" in schools, Canadian dance researchers Simon Barrick and his three colleagues[57] published a paper in 2012 that publicized the benefits to school boards and governments that dancing is significant for students' overall education.

For Ontario's students, they claim:

> [Dancing] helps to meet the needs of an ever increasingly diverse student population in that it offers alternative forms of instruction, learning, and assessment. This form of education should continue to become more prominent in order to meet Ontario's declining enrolment concerns.
>
> Dance within its own subject can become a way to reengage disenfranchised and marginalized students in personalized, meaningful learning methods.
>
> Dance allows students to construct their own knowledge and promotes the development of successful learning skills which will extend to postsecondary studies, the workplace, and beyond.

Dance professor Patricia Knowles adds that the outcome for students who dance is they would be "…touched by a sense of themselves as whole, moving, thinking, feeling, and culturally valued individuals."[58]

## Arrival of Eastern European Immigrant Dancers

Since 1605, immigration has played a vital role in developing Canada. During the second half of the twentieth century, liberal immigration policies encouraged newcomers while emphasizing multiculturalism. The federal government introduced a points-based system for evaluating applicants that resulted in a jump in immigrants from Africa, Asia, the Caribbean, and Latin America.

The 1990s and early 2000s were marked by the arrival of Eastern European immigrants with longstanding traditions of ballroom dancing. This influx of dancing talent was triggered by the 1991 collapse of the Union of Soviet Socialist Republics (USSR).

According to a study by David Outevsky on Soviet dancing talent being imported into Canada, the new arrivals from countries such as Ukraine, Georgia, Belarus, Armenia, Azerbaijan, Kazakhstan, Kyrgyzstan, Moldova, and Turkmenistan "were able to build significant cultural capital and establish a community base for themselves. As they settled in major cities in Canada, they imported their training methods and discipline ethics into the Canadian dance world."[59]

These methods were effective and resulted in the Soviet dancers eventually dominating the Canadian ballroom dance scene, said Outevsky.

## The 2014 Canada Dance Mapping Study

In 2011, Canada's public arts funder launched a comprehensive study to investigate the full nature of dancing in the country—the who, what, where, when, and why.

In its own words, the Canada Council for the Arts, in partnership with the Ontario Arts Council, said it wanted "to identify, quantify and describe the ecology, economy and environment of dance in Canada."[60]

Some highlights:
- Of the 8,124 respondents, 73% were leisure dance participants and 27% were dance professionals.

- Of the 190 dance forms represented, the two most common forms, "ballroom and social" as a single category was one of two most common forms of dance with 24%; the other was contemporary and modern dance (36%). As a proportion of all dance forms within the "ballroom and social" category, the breakdown was: ballroom 22%, lindy hop (12%), swing (12%), blues (8%), West Coast swing (7%), Balboa (4%), cha-cha (4%), and Charleston (4%).
- (Note to readers: Ballroom likely referred to International and American dance forms such as the two waltzes, quick step, foxtrot, rumba, jive, samba, swing, mambo, Peabody, etc.)
- 80% of survey respondents describe involvement in two to four forms of dance.[61]

The study also created a list of various dance organizations that support, among others, dance practitioners, dance educators, teachers and schools, recreational and participatory dancers, as well as participants in social dance.

Using some of the mapping study findings, dance journalist Lys Stevens produced a council research study on social dance and found that:

> A total of 571 social or participatory dance groups were identified across the country. These include square and round dance groups, Scottish country dancing groups, circle dancing, international and Israeli folk dance, swing clubs and other participatory dance groups.
>
> The majority of these fall under North American Dance. Some dance forms do not appear in this list that might have, such as salsa and tango, which were tabulated in relation to their annual events instead.[62]

## The New Ballroom Style

From the 1950s to the early 1970s, "club dancing" featuring contemporary music mixed with the favoured dances of the first seven decades of the twentieth century slowly became more dominant than traditional ballroom dancing.

Cal Pozo describes the changeover thus: "partner dancing, two people dancing as one, retreated to a handful of night clubs, ballroom dance halls and dance studios."[63]

However, the heyday of twist dancing in the sixties, along with seventies' disco dancing, paved the way for the more modern ballroom style, called the

English Style, later referred to as the International Style as people turned again to ballroom dancing for social reasons.

The first inkling of traditional ballroom evolving into modern ballroom occurred in 1812, when the waltz no longer was a set dance (that is, couples standing in a circle holding hands). "The dance form [then involved a] close proximity with which couples would dance, as well as the music that accompanied the dance."[64]

Some Canadian dance teachers, enthralled with this development, became spokespersons for the latest British experiment. Dance figures became codified and standards set for executing the figures that were based on a more natural way of moving.

Speaking to the American Society of Teachers of Dancing, Inc., at its ninetieth annual convention in 1957, Basil Valvasori, a Hamilton, Ontario-based instructor, recommended that Americans adopt the British style of ballroom dancing. The American group agreed with him, declaring that there was too much individuality on the ballroom floor.[65]

Valvasori declared the approach to the "standard" dances such as the slow waltz, Viennese waltz, quickstep, tango, and slow foxtrot should be:

> Certain rules must be followed at all times. There must always be bodily contact. At no time should you see space between man and the women. The partners should constantly look to the left.[66]

Many Canadian instructors accepted this new approach to social ballroom dancing. With this wide collective decision, they fundamentally changed social ballroom dancing forever—how it was taught and how it looked—and this change has sustained up to the twenty-first century.

However, strictly speaking, "social ballroom dancing" in Canada could no longer be called "social dancing," declared some dance experts. A clear explanation of why that was so came later. Juliet McMains, a former Canadian competitive (DanceSport) dancer and an assistant professor of dance at the University of Washington, explains:

> Dancing is something that in progress—active, alive, changing, and growing in the very moment of its execution. It is created and recreated by the practitioners each time they engage in the activity.
>
> Social ballroom dance [today] … contains little of this progressive energy, in which dancers themselves participate in creation of their own practice. Instead, it has more in common with *representations of social dance* [author's emphasis] on theatrical and

competition stages, with their emphasis on predetermined steps and precision of body lines.[67]

This view has yet to be challenged strongly by Canadian dance teachers. Since there has never been an association of *social* ballroom dancers or teachers to take up the cudgels for the view that social ballroom is not quite social dance due to its pre-determined choreography, it has remained an academic point.

McMains has always maintained that "the distinction I draw between these two categories is nuanced and has frequently been overlooked."

Provincial and national Canadian competitive dance associations have yet to comment on this distinction, since the issue is irrelevant to their aims and objectives.

## Social Dancing Becomes Popular Again Then Dips

From the late 1970s up to the turn of the century, there was a resurgence of social ballroom dancing in North America. The establishment of Golden Age clubs during this period in the earlier period led to more people, especially Canadian seniors, picking up the hobby to keep active.

Moncton, N.B. senior citizen Aurele Belliveau, speaking to a local newspaper reporter in 1999, jokingly claimed he did not need dance classes "because I thought I could dance already." He was one of tens of thousands of the grey-haired generation of people at the time whose life "has been defined by the romance of dance."[68]

For those starting a new journey in life, like starting a family, the "first dance" continued to be an important ritual at Canadian wedding receptions or post-wedding celebrations. For Rob and Cathy Kimball of London, Ontario, who got married in 1995, the tradition was significant, so much so that, according to *Chatelaine* magazine at the time, the couple seemed to be more focused on the choreography of their wedding dance and less on their Cape Cod honeymoon plan.

"All I could think abut was making it through our dance," said the bride.[69]

Many "first dances" in Canada since the beginning of the twenty-first century have been "social dance" based on prearranged dance figures. Called choreographic social dances, they are the staple of the many ballroom dance studios (listed in the appendix of the book) across the country.

The Arthur Murray Dance Centers and the Fred Astaire Franchised Dance Studios in Canada lead the pack, in terms of number of outlets, of private dance studios and municipal recreation departments in offering this type of dance service.

With this approach, students are taught a group of dance figures that are not leadable—which make it a much easier challenge for a couple to carry out. The two partners only need to memorize the same combination when practising and put them into effect.

The choreographic social dance approach is also the mainstay of the two groups of public providers of social dancing—the continuing education departments of school boards and the recreation departments of Canadian municipal governments.

In the immediate pre-COVID pandemic period, there has apparently been a decline in partner dancing, compared to two decades earlier. For those over fifty-plus especially, the change has to do with growing older.

The 30-year director of Toronto's West-Way Dance Club whose 500 members are mainly middle-aged plus, says it has been experiencing a gradual loss in attendance of its long-time dancers. "We had lots of couples that came before [I joined the club]. And then as they got older, we would lose them," Mary Fulton says.

When a member of a married couple passed away, "that almost ended the thing for the other person," she says. "Not all the time the [newly] single woman or a single man would show up. Some did, but some didn't."

Although the full extent of the drop in numbers by different age groups across the country is not known, it may be viewed as part of a cyclical pattern of highs and lows that has long been the country's experience. Various crosscurrents of changes in Canadian society brought about by technology, upheavals in gender roles and family relations are to blame.

In technology, the unintended consequences of phone or computer-based video calls, for example, in which a person can converse with others in real time have had an impact on interpersonal relations. B.C. dance instructor and blogger George Pytlik explains that "… people increasingly connect with each other through technology and are not so dependent on being together physically. When they do meet in person, they are more likely to seek out a bar or restaurant than a dance venue."[70]

Pytlik also attributes the current—and temporary, likely—change in interest in partner dancing to the negative effects of dancing competitions on the psyche of a lot of men. The *Dancing with the Stars* TV show that started in 2005—and is scheduled to launch its thirtieth season in 2021-2022—has created expectations among some men that they have to be able to dance like the male performers on the show.

This does not mean, however, that Canadian night clubs or the resorts in

Negril Jamaica have not been seeing multitudes of young male gyrating bodies on the dance floor or on beaches. The fact is that in those places, men are into free-form, no-touch dancing. In contrast, the more popular and intimate partner dances such as salsa, social ballroom/Latin, Argentine tango involve men having to lead and the women to follow in traditional ballrooms or other dancing venues.

According to dance instructors, leading is not just about doing the steps reasonably well, but also about interacting with the partner in such a way that the man, as leader, can dance relatively smoothly with the other person.

But, as Pytlik explains, "[m]en who aren't confident in their ability to lead will not be comfortable on a dance floor. Developing that skill requires a man to be willing to fail in front of women, and to do that he must have a strong sense of self-worth as he learns to dance."[71]

## The COVID-19 Pandemic: Tales of Hope for Social Dancers

The world of social dance began a long stop-and-go period starting in March 2020 when the COVID-19 pandemic crippled the Canadian economy and life in general. Like most other areas of recreational activity, social dancing came to a standstill.

With varying levels of restrictions in place at different times in the provinces and territories, privately owned social dancing providers such as dancing schools, social dance venues (both volunteer-run and commercial), and publicly funded organizations such as municipal recreation departments shut their doors.

The shuttering of dance services created a financial crisis for most of the providers who lost dance revenues since the start of the pandemic.

In October 2020, Véronique Clément, director of Québec's Dance Education Network, told the media that 430 dance schools, including social ballroom, Argentine tango and salsa studios, were closed, and 130,000 students were without dance classes.[72]

To counter the revenue losses, she asked for financial assistance from the Québec government. In response, the province announced various programs, including emergency assistance for small and medium-sized businesses and the Canada Emergency Rent Subsidy.

Dance studio owners and instructors in other jurisdictions suffered an equal blow during the same month and lobbied their government, just like their Québec counterparts.

In Ontario, studios in four regional "hot spots" for COVID-19 (Toronto, Ottawa, York, and Peel regions), where most of the province's private dance services providers are located), were forced to shut down. This was announced as part of a modified Stage 2 lockdown ordered by the provincial government.

Urging the government to reopen studios, Ontarians signed a petition to Ontario Premier Doug Ford to lift its restrictions on dance studios and other small businesses. The argument the petitioners made was that it was unfair to lump "dance studios" as part of "adult fitness classes" that were perceived to be a major cause of spreading the virus.

On October 19, 2020, the government announced that owners of dance studios in Ontario's COVID-19 hot spots were allowed to reopen their businesses.

"All participants must be pre-registered and maintain at least two metres apart," tweeted Lisa MacLeod, the minister responsible for heritage, sport, tourism, and culture industries.[73]

Having been lobbied by the dance community on the same issue, the mayor of Canada's largest city was pleased. John Tory announced in a tweet:

> Glad provincial officers have found a way for dance studios to reopen in Toronto and other areas in modified stage 2. Thank you to [the] minister … for working on this issue and thank you to the residents who reached out to identify the need for a change.[74]

> Like Québec and other jurisdictions, the Ontario government, in partnership with the federal government, announced various financial assistance programs to help dance studios.

> Ontario, Québec, and other provincial and territorial jurisdictions again announced modified lockdowns through the first half of 2021.

Thanks to technological platforms for communicating video and audio such as the Zoom app, dance providers of all kinds rose to the challenge of becoming closed shops permanently.

In the fall of 2020, the volunteer-run Calgary Dance Club exhorted its members in an email:

> We're all dancing at home. Join us!

> Fitness facilities and in-person events may be suspended for a while, but we've got a whole collection of online dance classes

available for you to watch when you want, as often as you want.[75]

The executive board of Newfoundland's Memorial University Ballroom & Latin Dance Club went one step further: it addressed the sound quality issue common to virtual dance instruction by making available songs "to use with their own speakers if needed."[76]

To keep things running, Toronto's 30-Up Club, the West-Way Club, and scores of other volunteer-run social dance organizations across Canada produced videos or held in-person classes based on the varying provincial or territorial time and public safety measures.

In Ontario, for instance, *Ontario Regulation 546/20*, issued on 2 October 2020, decreed that teachers—whether community-run or private—would not be allowed to hold group classes with more than ten students. Dances or dance practices would be allowed, but attendance had to be restricted to ten participants including the person running the dance and the DJ (disc jockey).

Canadian dance studio owners and other dance services providers responded in different ways to the pandemic restrictions at various times of their operations. Here is a sample of their initial reactions reported in the media during the first sixteen months of the pandemic:

## The National Square and Round Dance Community

OTTAWA—The 2020–2022 board of directors of the Canadian Square and Round Dance Society cancelled in-person dance activities of their provincial federations until the pandemic was over.

(A federation board of directors coordinates the dance activities of associations of clubs located in various geographic areas.)

Hundreds of dance cancellation notices were posted on club websites, while the national society encouraged members to run virtual square dancing and other dances.

The society had been excited about holding its national convention in 2020 and 2021 but postponed it to 2022.

## Nunavut

CAMBRIDGE BAY—During the first month of the pandemic, a Cambridge Bay drumming group, called Huqqullaaqatigiit, came up with a new way to host its weekly drum dance. The meaning of the group is people who sing and dance, and it went live on Facebook in March 2020. Organizer Julia Ogina even delivered songbooks to homes to help families follow along.[77]

## British Columbia

VANCOUVER—Small private dance studios such as Cory Solomon's Dance 4U that trains students in salsa in downtown Vancouver followed B.C.'s safety guidelines, including antivirus cleaning procedures. Without a hitch, the studio team, Corey Solomon, Samia Massoud, and Jessica Sage, successfully ran wedding dance courses as well as their private and semiprivate (four-to-six-person) salsa classes.[78]

In August 2020, larger operators such as E&R Ballroom Studio offered six social ballroom dance level 1, five level 2, and 3 level 3 classes in the Greater Vancouver area and Vancouver Island.[79]

Besides running several short courses during the entire pandemic period in 2020, the student-run University of British Columbia Dance Club ran four separate weekly international ballroom classes in the fall of 2020 with instructors Joel Marasigan, Zillion Wong, and Kyryl Dudchenko.[80]

## Alberta

CALGARY—Leo Sato, popularly known in the city as "Supertanguero," and his partner Marina Gonzalez conducted small semiprivate Argentine tango classes at Raw Canvas Art Studio during fall 2020, while complying with provincial pandemic guidelines.[81]

## Saskatchewan

SASKATOON—During the pandemic, members of the BKS YXE, a dance club widely known for its bachata, kizomba, and salsa classes, were longing for summer dancing at the cultural area in River Landing in their downtown.

However, the pandemic struck and wiped out the possibility. The club executive sent out this plea: "We encourage people to still keep in contact with each other by phone or online. We would love to hear everyone's creative suggestions for how we can continue to interact and support each other and our collective love of dance while minimizing physical contact!"[82]

## Manitoba

WINNIPEG—The Salsa Explosion Dance Company had to cope with the continual changes in provincial pandemic protective guidelines. From September 2020, it was allowed to resume in-person salsa and bachata classes provided they started wearing masks.

In November, however, the province was coded "red" and all classes were cancelled. Its Facebook message: "… [W]e have decided to close our doors until further notice. Although it saddens us to put a pause on dancing together, we believe that this is the safest decision for the community at this time. We look forward to dancing together soon, and we promise to open our doors again as soon as possible."[83]

## Ontario

TORONTO—The 400-seat West-Way Club, which opened at least once following the March 2020 provincial lockdown, closed again on October 10, 2020 and did not reopen until 2021.[84] (It closed again with further provincial lockdowns.)

SHAKESPEARE—During non-lockdown days in 2020, Melody and Francois Vallerand ran two sessions, one at their house and the other at the Knights of Columbus Hall in Stratford, fifteen kilometres away.

At home, a maximum of three couples learned and practised figures with no hands-on instruction or partner-switching. Appropriate social distancing, wearing masks, and a dedicated, well sanitized washroom exclusively for student use were the protective measures the Vallerand Dance studio instructors put into place.

At the external venue, they hosted ten masked couples in a large room.

MISSISSAUGA—Seen as a "Happy Holidays" gift to dancers, Mandy Epprecht, principal of Mandy's Dance studio in Mississauga posted online in late fall five videos on Latin dancing, including a beginner salsa line dance video featuring *La Gozadera* ("good time") *Yin*.[85]

HORSESHOE VALLEY—In an attempt to bypass the novel coronavirus while keeping invitees safe, Ralph Price ran two "driveway jam" session at his home, ninety kilometres north of Toronto. A caller with the Canadian Olde Tyme Square Dance Association, Price described in a September 4, 2020 email how the events went:

For the first jam we had 7 fiddlers, a bass, a keyboard and an audience of 9. At the second we had 5 fiddlers, a bass, a keyboard, a guitar and an audience of 8. While we couldn't do any square dancing, people who came as a couple were able to get up and dance to the waltzes, foxtrots and pattern dances.

TORONTO—Aleksander Saiyan's Toronto Dance Salsa studio sent this message to its students: "We know that 2020 has been a difficult year for all of us." The studio, located in the North York area, turned to virtual classes and at the start of the 2020 winter offered a free opportunity. "To help you have an amazing night, where you can still dance, have fun and meet cool people … Come join us for a free weekly interactive virtual Merengue lesson." [86]

OTTAWA—Tiniko Natsvlichvili of Milonga Querida in Ottawa expressed hope during the pandemic lockdown in Ontario. She invited her Argentine *tangueros* and *tangueras* to "get together on Zoom and chat about the future of Ottawa tango. I think we can all agree that this experience will create a change, so let's shine a light on it and move forward with collective intention." [87]

SUDBURY—Dennis Harasymchuk and his team at the Ballroom Dance Studios in Sudbury advertised a twelve-week Latin line dance fusion course that started on September 21, 2020, "with precautions … in place." [88]

## Québec

LAVAL—Baila Productions Salsa Dance School with studios in Laval, Pointe-Claire, and Claire Île-Perrot, kept two-way communications with their dancers. In a message, the studio said, "In order to follow public health guidelines, we are currently closed. Leave us your contact information by sending us an email or by calling us and we will keep you informed."[89]

MONTREAL—The San Tropez Dance Centre in Montreal assured its dancers on its website that providing "…a fun and enjoyable atmosphere has always been our number one priority, and we thank our students for your loyalty. Together we will get thru this! See you on the dance floor." During the pandemic, it offered online classes—private and group classes on zoom.[90]

## New Brunswick

ROTHESAY—The KV Ballroom Dancing studio suspended all activities and stated, "Depending on circumstances, classes (modified for safety) may resume mid-fall 2020 or winter 2021."[91]

## Nova Scotia

HALIFAX—In anticipation of the pandemic petering out by spring of 2021, Michel Dubé, owner and head instructor of Dancing with Michel & Company in Halifax, posted a five-day schedule of classes for ballroom, salsa, and jive. In early 2021, he indicated on his website that the classes would begin later in 2021.[92]

The reactions of non-square dance students and diehard social dancers were mixed.

In interviews with the author, most respondents' reaction was one of great disappointment. Since dancers love to dance, if not regularly, the restrictions, particularly ones that required wearing masks and dancing by oneself, were unacceptable, they told him.

Some dancers were not content with other restrictions such as the cap on numbers allowed to dance in enclosed spaces. In early fall of 2020, the 30-Up Club in Toronto received a letter from a member that mentioned "great unhappiness with the club's decision to limit the number of dancers at any one time to ten."

The executive board, headed by club president Marjorie White, wrote, "This was done to keep us in compliance with new rules [by the Ontario government] for venues where there is dancing."

"We are dancing—with the attendant level of risk associated with dancing indoors. Your board of directors is not happy with scaled back regulations, but we have legal and fiduciary responsibilities to comply," the report said.[93]

The 30-Up Club used humour to help ease the anxiety that members felt around the pandemic. The club president's husband, Justin White, wrote several newsletters with the tagline "Dancing Around the Virus."

# Conclusion

The above history of social dancing, defined as dancing for pleasure and recreation, is only a sketch for a possible broader study that remains to be done.

One thing is certain about Canada's past social dancing activities: while the many dance forms Canadians love have changed—and are still evolving—we have traditionally turned to dancing as an avenue to express a range of emotions. These emotions represented a reaction to what had happened in society when Canada was both a French and English colony. Since Confederation in 1867, it continues to play an important part in the lives of Canadians.

The country's Indigenous peoples were the first dancers. Their multidimensional dancing traditions go back centuries—long before 1605 when the French colony of Canada was established with the first permanent settlement in Nova Scotia.

In this chapter, social dancing in all its forms has been shown to be a ritual that Canadians from all walks of life have practised to their mutual delight and unending joy.

It has also been about gender—how men and women have related to one another. As well, it is clear it has also been about the differences in wealth and prestige and the feelings and attitudes about social class and status.

Up to the middle of 2021, when this book was written, the COVID-19 pandemic was still upending the recreational dancing activities of Canadians. When it appears in the rear-view mirror, so to speak, there will likely be an explosion of dancing—social and competitive—across the country to release the pent-up demand for emotional expression and bodily movement to music.

---

[1] Warren E, Kalbach, "Population of Canada," *The Canadian Encyclopedia*, accessed 23 April 2020.
[2] Iro Tembeck. "Dancing in Montréal: seeds of a choreographic histpry," *The Journal of the Society of Dance History Scholars*, vol. 5, no.2, fall 1994, p1.
[3] Juliet McMains, op.cit., p.67. A.H. Franks, op. cit., p.168.
[4] Theresa Jill Buckland, "From the artificial to the natural body: social dancing in Britain, 1900-1914," in Eds. Alexandra Carter & Rachel Fensham. *Dancing Naturally: nature, neo-classicism and modernity in early twentieth-century dance*. London: Palgrave Macmillan, 2011.
[5] McMains, op.cit., p.71.
[6] Ibid. pp.66-67.
[7] Ted Tjaden. "Ragtime music in Canada:. http://www.ragtimepiano.ca/rags/can2.htm, accessed 30 July 2020.

[8] Ellen Arual, Canada's entertainment in the 1920s, https://772708911112410211.weebly.com/contact.html accessed 15 November 2020.

[9] Fred Daugherty. "The 'animal dancers' so wild they were banned from the White House: When a 'turkey trot' craze swept the nation in the 1910s, authority figures panicked". https://www.history.com/news/banned-animal-dance-turkey-trot-woodrow-wilson, accessed 19 November 2020.

[10] Gray Miller. "History of social dance." Lovetoknow Corp. Burlingame, CA. https://dance.lovetoknow.com/History_of_Social_Dance accessed 2 Dec. 2020.

[11] McMains, op.cit., p.82

[12] P. o'D. "Taking the tang out of tango," *Saturday Night*, 13 December 1913, p.6.

[13] Anon. Letter. "Advice to girls," *The Daily Mail*. St. John's., Newfoundland, 18 March 1914.

[14] McMains, Juliet, op.cit., p.112.

[15] There were "state balls" in 1904, 1907, 1908, and 1912. These were invitational entertainments with dinner and dancing attended by local elites as well as high-level invitees from Montréal and other cities and towns and hosted by the Governors-General.

[16] Anonymous. "Tango not permitted at Rideau Hall ball," *The Globe*, 9 December 1913, p.1.

[17] Ibid.

[18] Carissa Wong. "The roaring twenties." https://medium.com/@wong_carissa/the-roaring-twenties-13d375bb4085, accessed 3 December 2020.

[19] Cheryl M. Willis, *Tapping the Apollo: the African American female tap dance duo salt and pepper*. Jefferson, N.C.: MCFarland & Company, Inc., 2016.

[20] Anonymous. "History of radio broadcasting. In Canada." History of broadcasting in Canada - Wikipedia, accessed 22 November 2020.

[21] Ted Magder, Piers Handling and Peter Morris. "Canadian Film History: 1896 to 1938." *The Canadian Encyclopedia* https://www.thecanadianencyclopedia.ca/en/article/the-history-of-film-in-canada, accessed 30 September 2020.

[22] Anonymous. "Canada's entertainment in the 1920s" https://prezi.com/hb5dzkksh_zgp/canadas-entertainment-in-the-1920s/#:~:text=Dances%20such%20as%20the%20charleston.%2C%%20and%20Lindy%20Hop

[23] Anonymous. "Montréal in roaring twenties." https://www.canadahistory.ca/explore/arts-culture-society/toot-sweet-when-jazz-ruled-Montréal, accessed 6 July 2020.

[24] Brianna FitzHenry. "1920s Canada." https://1920sentertainmentbybrianna.weebly.com/jazz-and-other-music.html, accessed 2 December 2020.

[25] Mark Knowles, op.cit., p.174.

[26] Richard Powers, https://socialdance.stanford.edu/Syllabi/jazz_age.htm, accessed 3 August 2020.

[27] Mary Jane Warner, op.cit.

[28] Standards for dancing were motivated by several factors, all interacting with one another: (a) The freewheeling improvisation by couples for the new dances needed to be halted, according to dancing analysts. As a commodity, dancing—and the marketing of it—had to sustain class status. (b) The English dance authorities, viewing with horror the wildness of Americans dancing when U.S. soldiers visited Europe during the First World War, moved quickly to distance the dances from their low-class Afro-American roots, according to the dance scholar Danielle Anne Robinson at Toronto's

Ryerson University. "[T]hose performing the 'refined' modern dances were distancing themselves from the black creative innovators of these dances." (Juliet McMains, op.cit., paraphrasing a thesis in Robinson's Ph.D. diss., "Race in motion: reconstructing the practice, profession and politics of social dance." University of California, Riverside, 2004.)

29 Anonymous. "New styles influenced by dances." *The Toronto World,* 13 January 1914, vol. XXXIV, no. 12, p.216.

30 Ibid.

31 "Great depression in Canada," https://en.wikipedia.org/wiki/Great_Depression_in_Canada, accessed 5 October 2020.

32 Katrina Srigley. *Breadwinning daughters: young working women in a depression-era city, 1929-1939,* Toronto: University of Toronto Press, 2010, pp.99-100,

33 The Canadian Press. "Bad for discipline: women teachers must not teach boy students dancing," *The Globe,* 13 December 1935, p.1.

34 Ibid., p.119.

35 Helen McNamara. "Dance bands," https://www.thecanadianencyclopedia.ca/en/article/dance-bands-emc, accessed 7 Sept. 2020.

36 Katrina Srigley, op.cit., p. 123.

37 Peter Young. *Let's dance: a celebration of Ontario's dance halls and summer dance pavilions.* Toonto: Natural Heritage/Natural History Inc., 2002, p.iii.

38 Catherine Gidney. "The Dredger's daughter: courtship and marriage in the Baptist community of Welland, Ontario, 1934-1944." *Labour (*Committee on Canadian Labour History), pp.121-149.

39 Lisa Doolittle. "The Trianon and on: reading mass social dancing in the 1930s and 1940s in Alberta, Canada." *Dance Research Journal,* Winter 2001, vol.33, no. 2.

40 *The Vancouver Sun,* https://www.newspapers.com/image/?clipping_id=35351241&fcfToken=eyJhbGciOiJIUzI1NiIsInR5cCI6IkpXVCJ9.eyJmcmVlLXZpZXctaWQiOjQ5MDU0MTk2NywiaWF0IjoxNjA2NzUyMjQ3LCJleHAiOjE2MDY4Mzg2NDd9.FujAW92ZlpDz_-HnMYDoD7B-Pp-QFU_Bk5jARcZybRE

41 John Mackie, "This week in history, 1938: Vancouver's first music star returns home to play the hotel Vancouver," *Vancouver Sun,* 21 October 2016. https://vancouversun.com/news/local-news/this-week-in-history-1938-vancouvers-first-music-star-returns-home-to-play-the-hotel-vancouver/, accessed 23 January 2021.

42 Anonymous. "Sunny Fry Orchestra engaged for board of trade dance," *Bassano Recorder,* 4 April 1940, p.1, Bassano Recorder (ualberta.ca)

43 Joy-Ann Cohen. "Last waltz played by old time band," *The Leader-Post,* 11 March 1977, p.10.

44 Anonymous. "Duke Ellington and His Orchestra setlist" Duke Ellington & His Orchestra Concert Setlist at Trianon Ballroom, Regina on June 29, 1954 | setlist.fm

45 Anonymous. *The Lethbridge Telegram,* 15 January 1918.

46 *The Wetaskiwin Times,* 19 January 1922, Item A100416, p.4.

47 Iro Tembeck. "Dancing in Montreal: seeds of a choreographic history," *The Journal of the Society of Dance History Scholars,* vol. 5, no. 2, Fall 1994.

48 Gerald Hallowell. "Prohibition in Canada," *The Canadian Encyclopedia.* Prohibition in Canada | The Canadian Encyclopedia

49 Jessica Herdman. *The Cape Breton fiddling narrative: Innovation, preservation, dancing.* M.A. Thesis, University of British Columbia, August 2008, p.89.

50 Ibid.

51 Dan Malleck. *Try to control yourself: The regulation of public drinking in post-Prohibition Ontario 1927-44*, Vancouver: University of British Columbia, 2013. p.137.

52 Ibid.

53 Please see Richard Powers' "Teen dances of the 1950s" for a detailed coverage of 1950s dancing. Teen Dances of the 1950s (stanford.edu)

54 See Richard Powers, op.cit. 1970s Disco Dances (stanford.edu) for a detailed look at these dances.

55 David Outevsky. *Soviet bodies in Canadian dancesport: cultural identities, embodied politics, and performances of resistance in three Canadian ballroom dance studios*. PhD. Diss., Toronto: York University, 2018, p.104.

56 Albertson, Karen. http://www.jointhedance.com/testimonials.php

57 Simon Barrick, Lindsay Kavanaugh, Keith Macfarlane, and Theodore Christou. *The history of dance education in 20th century Ontario schools: 1950 to 2010.* 19 November 2012. https://www.curriculumhistory.org/Studies_in_Curriculum_History_and_Educational_Philosophy/Select_Subjects_in_the_History_of_Ontario_Education_files/The%20History%20of%20Dance%20Education%20in%2020th%20Century%20Ontario%20Schools.pdf

58 Patricia Knowles. "Dance education in American public schools," *Bulletin of the Council for Research in Music Education*, Summer, 1993, no. 117, p.46.

59 David Outevsky, op.cit., p.103.

60 "Summary of the Canada Dance Mapping Study." Canada Council for the Arts 1 December 2016, Summary of the Dance Mapping Study | Canada Council for the Arts

61 EKOS Research Associates Inc. *Summary: findings from Yes I Dance : a survey of who dances in Canada: bringing the arts to life.* (Canada Council for the Arts, 21 July 2014 Executive_Summary_Yes_I_Dance_EN.pdf

62 Lys Stevens. *Dancing across the land: a report on the Canada Dance Mapping Inventory: bringing the arts to life* (Canada Council for the Arts) 30 July 2013. file:///C:/Users/John/Downloads/140520-Inventory-EN.pdf

63 Cal Pozo, *Let's dance: the complete book and DVD of ballroom dance instruction for weddings, parties, fitness and fun*. Long Island City, N.Y.: Harleigh Press, 2007.p.xv.

64 Sarah Godel. "Ballroom: the dance that globalization built." Ballroom: The Dance That Globalization Built « Interrogating Dance Globalization (smith.edu)

65 The Canadian Press, "U.S. society recommends British style of dancing," *The Globe and Mail*, 6 August 1957, p.18.

66 Ibid.

67 Juliet McMains, op,cit. p.64.

68 Cathryn Spence. "For the love of dance: Aurele Bellivea's life has been defined by the romance of dance," The (Moncton) *Times-Transcript*, 25 June 1999.

69 Janice Biehn, "Let's dance," *Chatelaine* (English ed.), December 1995.

70 George Pytlik, "Has there been a decline in ballroom dancing. Why[?] https/www/quora/com.Has-there-been-a-decline-in-ballroom-dancing-why/, accessed 2 September 2020.

71 Ibid.

72 Global News. https://globalnews.ca/news/7406718/coronavirus-Québec-dance-academies/, accessed 23 October 2020

73 Lisa MacLeod. (20) Lisa MacLeod (@MacLeodLisa) / Twitter

74 Ibid.

75 The Calgary Dance Club. Email to members. 28 November 2020.
76 MUN Ballroom & Latin Dance Club, https://www.facebook.com/groups/6027805871/.
77 CBC News. "Nunavut drumming group finds new way to get together, despite physical distancing." 3 March 2020. https://www.cbc.ca/news/canada/north/cambridge-bay-drumming-group-nunavut-connection-1.5517015
78 COVID-19 – Dance 4U Salsa, Bachata, Swing and Wedding Dance Lessons (dance4uvancouver.com)
79 E & R Ballroom Dance *Newsletter for Sunday November 22nd* 2020. E & R Ballroom Dance eandrballroomdance.com
80 UBC Dance Club. *http://ubcdanceclub.com/online-classes/*
81 Leo Sato's Premier Argentine Tango School. TangoCalgary.com – Leo's Tango Calgary Website
82 BKSYXE Let's Dance (Studio) *https://bksyxe.ca/*
83 Salsa Explosion Dance Company. https://www.facebook.com/salsaexplosiondancecompany/ 2 November 2020.
84 The West-Way Club. https://thewestwayclub.ca/
85 30-Up Club. Listserve@30-up.com 21 October 2020
86 Toronto Dance Salsa. Toronto. https://torontodancesalsa.ca/free5095/
87 Milonga Querida. Ottawa: *https://www.facebook.com/MilongaQueridaOttawa/*
88 Ballroom Dance Studios. Sudbury, ON. http://ballroomdancestudios.ca
89 Bailar Productions. West Perth, ON. *https://www.bailarproductions.com/dance*
90 Latindance.net. Montréal: https://www.latindance.net/language/en/health-safety/
91 KV Ballroom Dancing (Studio) Ottawa: https://www.kvballroomdancing.com
92 Dancing with Michel & Company. Halifax, N.S.:http://dancingwithmichel.ca/schedule.shtml
93 30-Up Club, op.cit.

# Chapter 2: Having the Time of Their Social Dancing Life!

I'm online every morning at 8 a.m., then I take a break to go dance, and then I'm back online by 10. When I return, I feel more awake, juicier and more creative. The world looks brighter to me. I feel more ready to meet the day, whether that involves work or childcare or being there for my friends. This pandemic is a marathon. But taking the time to dance every day feels like hitting a reset button. I'm able to start each day fresh." — Rebekah Blok in an interview with Isabel B. Slone in *Toronto Life* magazine, Dec. 31, 2020

99% of all dance students will never perform on a stage, but 100% will have to dance at a wedding or other function. — Chris Thorburn, owner, Kelowna Ballroom, B.C..[1]

## Living and Dancing

Imagine a dystopian Canada!

A Canada in which men and women, boys and girls are banned from dancing—alone or with others. In other words, a world in which people are denied access to pleasurable sensations by moving to music.

In such a suppressed world, millions of non-dancers would never again be able, from the side of a ballroom hall or on TV, to see a pivoting salsa dancer or four pairs of either modern or "olde tyme" square dancers doing a "roll away to a half sashay." Nor would they be able to enjoy the artsy movements of towering social ballroom dancers or Argentine *tangueros* and *tangueras*.

What could be an even worse situation: a newly married beautiful bride and her husband not allowed to do their first dance!

But the reality—except for the COVID-19 pandemic period from March 2020 to sometime in 2021 perhaps—happens to be the opposite.

Any day outside of work, twisting and twirling bodies move around while rhythmic music prevails. Across the vast Canadian landscape, in urban dance halls, social clubs, dance studios, community centres, school gyms, barns, and home kitchens, plenty of people are dancing for recreation.

In some of those places, you might also find curious onlookers.

The dancers' moves may not look perfect, like on episodes of *Dancing with the Stars*, but for them, whatever they execute does wonders for them. There are smiles galore, romantic eyes glowing. Occasionally, some dancers might step on each other's toes, provoking a "Sorry!" and "It's OK."

Mississauga, Ontario, salsa dancer Gregory Evelyn confesses he does not always learn a new dance figure right away, like other student *salseros* (people who dance salsa). "I may end up being bad at it for a while," Gregory says, "but I'm OK with that."

But when he finally grasps it, he is extremely happy. "[Also] I'm doing something that I enjoy, and getting that benefit … feeling more confident," he says.

For twenty something Torontonian Arkady Silverman, who has been doing international-style ballroom dancing since she was nine, doing the moves she's learned for more than a decade is all about "… a freedom of movement, freedom of body, and also a flow to the body."

The good feelings the Toronto-based university research assistant experiences through dancing sometimes extend to breakfast time. "I will dance [by myself] while getting ready in the morning and while brushing my teeth. I'd [even] dance around the kitchen while cooking.…" Silverman explains.

Back in 2015, when he was facing a body-balancing challenge, Calgary retiree Tadahiro Okazawa started do less mountaineering, skiing, and sailing and took up Argentine tango.

"I'm enjoying it very much," he says. "Initially, it was very intimidating; every man [in my classes] looked so advanced … and I feared no lady would like to dance with me," says Tadahiro. "On the contrary, most were kind and willing to dance at least one *tanda* (a set of music pieces played in a turn of dancing that lasts about 10 minutes) with me."

Today, he and his regular tango partner, Louise McKay, regularly attend *milongas* (social events for Argentine tango dancers).

Beginner-level dancers who practise specific figures in a set manner will usually acquire the confidence they need for the next skill level, say dance instructors.

And that's exactly what Louise and Tadahiro's strategy has always been: they always dance the first and last *tandas*—although they dance with others at social dance events.

"We feel we have gotten better by doing it this way as it becomes a specific pattern if you only dance with your partner, and you end up doing the same thing over and over," McKay declares.

A Vancouver-based paramedic at BC Emergency Health Services, Ying Cheung strives every day to balance out the stress levels that come with his job. With social dancing, badminton, and volleyball, in that order, he has found a lifeline. Starting with the West Coast swing, salsa, bachata and hip-hop dances while still in high school, Cheung went on, in 2018, to international ballroom dancing with the UBC (University of British Columbia) Dance Club.

Early in 2020, he spent many hours practising with a partner and staying on after classes to ask instructors for help in executing techniques. "I was at my high point in dancing two days before the UBC Gala Ball [cancelled in March 2020 due to the COVID-19 pandemic]. I was feeling confident about all my dances," Yeung recalls. "I was in a good spot."

Unlike the protagonist in Lewis Carroll's famous 1865 novel,[2] Alice Meinecke does not have to go to subterranean caves near Bracebridge in Ontario to discover a new world. Meinecke and her four girlfriends (she called them "the group of five" until the eldest of them passed away) are quick to carpool to the nearest place where fiddle music is in the air and fellow square-dancer gentlemen are waiting. She adds that there are 30 square and round dancing clubs south of Bracebridge, a town 170 kilometres north of Toronto.[3]

Another dancing adventure for fifty-something Meinecke is the biannual Toronto square dance festival. "When you go in," she says, "[there is] the opportunity to learn brand new dance patterns that aren't typically done" where she lives—a three-hour drive south.

"That is always just so much fun there ... new callers (the person who prompts the dance patterns), new dances. You know what the fun the whole evening is going to be," she says.

# Social Dancers' Thoughts on Their Passion and Art

In the years immediately preceding the COVID-19 pandemic period of the twenty-first century, partnered dancing has been popular in the Canadian "public culture," although probably not as much as at the beginning of the millennium.

There is overwhelming proof that social dancing elicits changes in the mood of those who participate in it. People sense a heightened mind-body connection. Overall, dancing arouses positive energy, according to dance instructors and students.

Below are mini accounts of social dancers from all walks of life—from all corners of Canada, expressing their thoughts during interviews with the author during 2020 and 2021 about their dancing.

# What It Really Means

### Ying Cheung in Vancouver and social ballroom/Latin

In Toronto, it is Salsa on St. Clair, a summer event each year that attracts hundreds of salsa dancers along a major road for two large city blocks, gyrating to scintillating music from live bands.

Vancouver's equivalent to the Toronto event is the Robson Square Summer Dance Series, and the West coast city's dance event is longer, every Friday night, June through early September.

As the Friday summer afternoons in Vancouver melt into the warm evenings, Ying can be spotted near the corner of Robson and Howe in the downtown core behind the Vancouver Art Gallery.

A free lesson, social dancing, and demonstrations from local dance stars are a huge draw for him and dozens of his colleagues, including Juliana Chow, a former president of the University of British Columbia Dance Club, and her former executive members.

According to DanceSport BC, organizers of the event, the annual event attracts some 800 dancers. "It's a very social, very inviting environment," says Ying. "Whenever I go there to dance, I just have fun.

"There are dancers of all levels dancing together, and [it's so crowded] I have to really think about where I need to go when I am dancing and what steps to be able to dodge the huge crowd of people swirling around me," says Ying.

## Vivian Brailean in Moose Jaw, Saskatchewan, and square dancing

For retiree Vivian, joining the square-dancing fraternity in the province's fourth largest city has been one of the best things she has embarked on. "The sociability of it … I met so many people … every square dancer [I've met] has become a friend." In 2021, she served on the eight-person executive of Zone 5 of the Saskatchewan Square & Round Dance Federation.

## Dorothy Campbell and partner in Saskatoon, Saskatchewan. and square dancing

Dorothy is a square dancer, as well as a diehard advocate and volunteer worker for the square-dancing cause for Zone 3 (Saskatoon) of the Saskatchewan Square & Round Dance Federation. As a zone representative, she is editing the newsletter and compiling a province-wide directory while dancing as much as she can.

But it took a while before she arrived at that point.

She and her partner first started dancing in the 1970s but left the square dance scene, although they had "a good time" and took up bowling for the following fourteen years. They were much younger then and thought initially they were in the wrong place, she said.

When we looked around the square, everybody was older than us," she recalls. "We felt this was for older people."

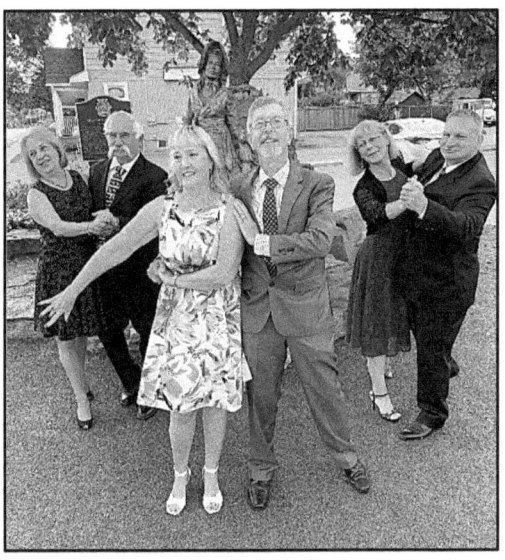

Figure 3: Statue of Elizabeth Posthuma Simcoe, née Gwillim in Bradford West Gwillimbury, Ontario: Three Bradford ballroom dancing couples pose near the statue (in the background) in a local parkette. Mrs Simcoe's diaries contain many references to her dancing at eighteenth century balls. (Exactly two hundred and nine years ago on Sept. 12, 2000 when this photo was taken, her husband, John Graves Simcoe, began his term in 1791 as first Lieutenant-Governor of Upper Canada, present day Ontario.) Photo shows, from left to right, Ginette Kanyo, John Kanyo, Eleanor Dyke, Dean Little, Nella Keating and Patrick Keating.

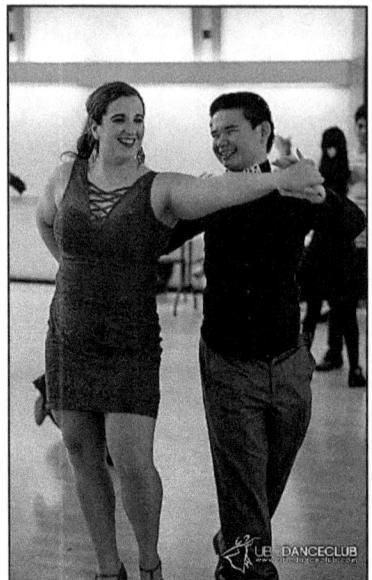

Figure 4: Social dancers Timothy Tan and Theresa Bodnarchuk dancing one evening at the University of British Columbia Dance Club in Vancouver.

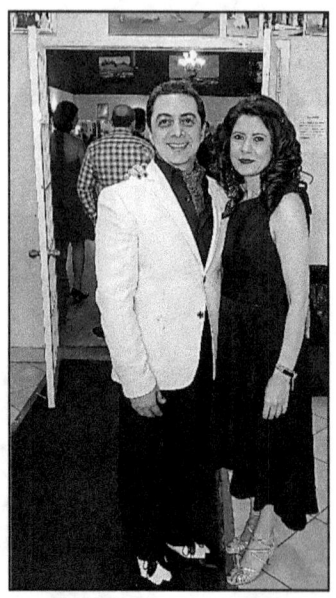

Figure 5: Dressed up in their spiffy dance outfits, dancers Torontonians Minoo Asgary and Omar Kazi get ready to enter their favourite dance hall.

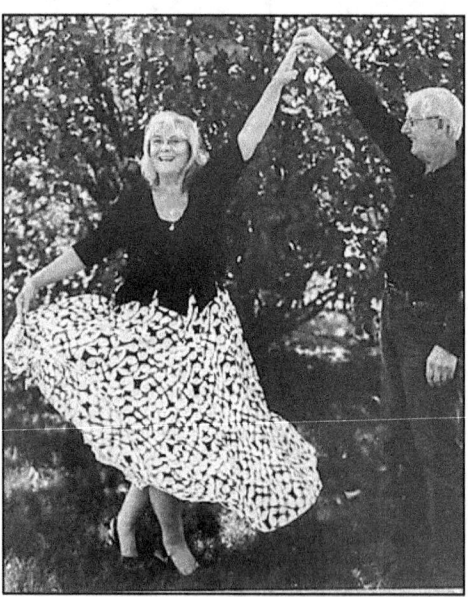

Figure 6: Bill Gibzey and Flori Mackie dance outdoors in Bradford West Gwillimbury, ON.

## Nella and Patrick Keating in Bradford–West Gwillimbury, Ontario, and social ballroom/Latin

Long before they retired from their jobs as computer information specialists in Ontario Hydro, Patrick and Nella mulled over some ideas to do something together that was outside the home and "fun".

According to Patrick, it had to be "some form of physical activity that would guarantee what we were going to be doing once a week."

Social ballroom dancing at one of Bradford–West Gwillimbury, Ontario, community centres in the 2000s turned out to be "really, really enjoyable, learning figures and keeping your mind going and a challenge to learn something," he remembers.

"You know," adds Nella, "we formed a lot of new friendships through dancing, and some of them are our great friends."

## Eleanor Dyke and Dean Little in Bradford–West Gwillimbury and social ballroom/Latin

Eleanor recently put away her colour wheel, paint chips, and fabric samples so she can follow her passion for dancing with more fervour.

The former Bradford–West Gwillimbury interior designer wants to dance more with her partner because she is enjoying her dance classes in her town that she says are "lots of fun and informative.

"I feel I'm on cloud nine when Dean and I are dancing," Eleanor beams with enthusiasm.

Dancing "has given me a more enriched social life through a wider circle of people I've met," says Dean. "The exercise I get has increased; I am better physically coordinated, and that I need at my age."

Deans says dancing "pushes you to interact with your partner a lot, a lot more than any other kinds of activities," echoing the sentiments of many other dancers.

## Jeanette and John Kanyo in Bradford–West Gwillimbury and social ballroom/Latin

For Jeanette and John, dancing has opened new vistas in socializing. After they started taking dance classes more than a decade ago, social dance events have assumed a greater meaning beyond the dancing itself.

When he and Jeanette go out, "You're not walking in on strangers. You see people you know, and they wave and say, 'Hi, how are you'?" John notes.

"Whether at the buffet tables or wherever, you can stop and shoot the breeze with them—it's kind of nice," he adds.

Jeanette says dancing has been a boon to her life, especially since she is now retired. "I find dancing relaxing," she says. "A new world opened up for me and John ... the people we've met in dances have been wonderful."

As for the overall effect of taking dance classes, John says, "It's nice when you're able to take lessons, and then you can go to venues with confidence because you know real dance steps, instead of jumping around.

"I think you'd be more comfortable on the dance floor if you know some real dance figures."

Since they started dance classes, the Kanyos have befriended a particular group. Their friendship with this group has blossomed to the extent that they sometimes go to New Year's Eve dance celebrations together. To top it all off, they have even taken a boat cruise together and visited Europe.

## Dale and J.J. Lubberts in East Gwillimbury, Ontario, and social ballroom/Latin

J.J. is clear about how dancing has changed his life. When he started dancing later in life, "It felt like opening the door of a room and not knowing what's behind the door," he says.

"When I opened it, there was a whole room of discoveries, things I didn't know, and the dancing was it."

Describing herself as "very shy about many things," Dale says going to the dance floor was "a confidence-builder, that also helped me in speaking in public.

"It's very hard, very difficult to feel sad or to be in a bad mood when you're dancing and listening to beautiful music.

"It's like going on a beach for a walk and listening to the waves. It's got that sort of calming, beautiful thing for me—it's both fun and energizing," she says.

## Jacinta Willems in Mitchell, Ontario, and Argentine tango

After a trip to Cuba in the early 2010s, Jacinta rediscovered dancing after a long lull due to her studies and work life in natural healthcare. Salsa was the stimulus. Despite the scintillating sounds of the music and the vibrant energies it ignited, however, she felt a "deeper longing in my soul that needed to find expression."

She turned to Argentine tango and found it "an expression of the feminine," as she puts it. "Tango for me is going very deep in a receptive state" that she has also found in meditation.

For Jacinta, the point is the tango is not just about dancing but also "complete surrender and trust and becoming very aware of oneself at a kinesthetic level."

## Karen Paton-Evans and Jim Evans in Shakespeare, Ontario, and social ballroom/Latin

After tying the knot in 1988, the Evans saw dancing as a way "to make real time for each other as a couple."

"We decided we needed to schedule something that would become a regular date night for us," explains Karen. "We figured some type of class or something would probably be best. So I said to Jim, well, I leave it up to you, whatever you want, to sign us up for a class."

Soon after, upon learning about their future dance instructors, François and Melody Vallerand, who teach at the Victoria Park Community Centre in the town of Ingersoll, Jim turned to Karen and declared, "Let's go ballroom dancing, Karen."

The rest is history.

## Maria Dobrynina and Alex Dobrynin in Newmarket, Ontario, and social ballroom/Latin

On many Wednesday nights, Maria and Alex have always been in a rush to get to the Armitage Village Public School in Newmarket to catch their dance class at 7:30 p.m.

When they return home from work on Wednesdays, the dance class has been a sort of lifeline as it provides "a great way to improve our quality of life, improve our self-confidence and boost our memory and physical coordination."

Turning to look at Alex, she says, "I can't leave out the fact that practising dancing with my husband has brought much fun and romance."

## Diane Ternan and David Franks in Newmarket and social ballroom/Latin

"It's a very pleasant way of making contact with each other in a crowd and enjoying music," says David, referring to his and his life partner's participation in the social dance classes in Newmarket, Ontario, several years ago.

Retired in 2020, David declares that to dance "is to enter a very different world. It's very intense, it's being very focused on each other. It's focused on the gift of music."

"It's fun, it's expressing the joy and power of music of the planet and connecting with each other," Diane adds.

Explaining the power of personal connection engendered by dancing, David says when he and Diane go sailing on his father's dinghy or go biking or camping together, "the focus is, sort of, on the nature around us rather than on the interaction between us."

## Sandra Holliday-Tucker and Silas ("Sie") Tucker in Newmarket and social ballroom/Latin

Sie is quick to credit social ballroom dancing with the healing of a serious leg injury sustained when he was thirteen years old.

Going to a gym, which he considers "boring," would not have done the trick. However, going to a dance class is "actual fun" and "you learn how to dance and dancercise at the same time."

In fact, the sixty something dancer is an example of "dance movement therapy" doing good.

In addition to the general mental and emotional benefits of dancing, Sie has reconnected with his life and dance partner, Sandra, in a big way.

"I find that getting out there and doing the lessons—and even doing the social dancing—makes me happier," Sandra says. "There's the emotional satisfaction and there's that sense of satisfaction when pushing yourself a little bit to learn something new.

"It's always really nice when you get that step and remember that little bit of a routine," she adds. "It's an amazing sense of satisfaction."

The Newmarket couple also associates their moving together in unison with music—and even moving past missteps—as a "personal performance" and an artistic expression to feel good about.

Sometimes when she is dancing with Sie at the Toronto's West-Way Club, she feels they "actually hit all of the points of a good presentation," like the tilt of the body and holding the head properly.

## Liboire (a.k.a. Lee) Brossard in Montréal and salsa

For former Torontonian Lee, who now lives in Montréal, a key part of salsa dancing is enjoying the dance and being selfless: "It's getting to the lady partners to attain a different level of feeling about how they are dancing. It's bringing out the best in them," he explains. "When you can see them smile and you can lead them to move … it's amazing."

Adds Lee, "The big thing about dancing is to be more present with the partner, because it's really not so much about you—it's about the woman in the picture frame."

## Esther and Barry Stanfield in Saint-Bruno, Québec and square dancing

Esther and her husband, a former university professor of physics, have been square dancing in their spare time.

They sometimes join their friends at the Swinging Stars, a Montréal area dance group that plays a wide repertoire of music, including rock 'n' roll, country, western, Caribbean, Irish, polkas, and oldies.

Although Barry is now retired, his declining ear health limits his ability to hear musical beats at dances.

But this does not stop them from attending dances. She is still as enthusiastic about dancing as she was when she was younger. "When I was a child and going home to my grandmother, I would put away my books," she says. "And then I would dance in the middle of the rice fields."

As an adult, she says dancing "makes me feel great. It's something to look forward to and to enjoy.

"I feel euphoric when I'm dancing. I don't need drugs. I just need music, and I dance in the kitchen, in the bedroom, I dance downstairs."

## Cristina Chirca in Montréal and salsa

"It's kind of a therapy for me," says Latin Groove's salsa dance instructor, Cristina. "When I'm dancing, nothing else matters. Nothing else actually exists. I am in the moment."

The former social and competitive ballroom dancer says "worries are not a problem when I am dancing—they just magically disappear … and that's how it becomes therapy.

"It becomes a drug … you're constantly seeking the feeling of pureness."

## Kathryn Stone in Halifax, Nova Scotia and Argentine tango

After four years into dancing tango, Kathryn says, "I love the community … we have a lovely community here in Nova Scotia. One of the most enjoyable moments I've had is when I'm really working my brain."

While dancing prolifically as a follower, she is upping her game by working on the leader's part—a step usually considered as stepping-stone to teaching in the future. But learning to lead is not only challenging, it has also led to her sliding into moments in which "I felt being in the flow state and having the most enjoyable moments."

## Vaunda and Martin Vanderaa in Charlottetown, Prince Edward Island, and square dancing

When Vaunda and Martin are not fielding calls from fellow P.E.I. square dancers about the dance events, she and Martin make time to be active as event planners in the Charlotte Twirlers, the only square dance club in the province. "It's a nice group of people to hang around with for exercise … and with the music thrown in, it just makes us feel good," says Vaunda. "Everybody is always very welcoming and friendly."

# Getting Started on the Journey

## Merv Meyer in Kamloops, British Columbia, and square dancing

Sitting in an Abbotsford bar a few decades ago was a fateful evening for Merv. Invited by a lady, a stranger, to go to a Thursday night square dance, he decided to attend the event, and according to him, "I've never looked back."

At the time, he was a heavy-duty mechanic. Today he is a square dance caller and teacher at Thompson Valley Stars (TV Stars), having started his teaching career in 1994.

TV Stars consists of Merv and his wife, Sandy-Gregson Meyer, whom he met in square dance circles. They call, cue, and teach "Mainstream &

Plus" and two-step waltz, rumba, cha-cha-cha and jive round dancing. They are members of the Thompson-Shuswap Square & Round Dance Association in Region 9 of the B.C. Square & Round Dance Federation.

## Vivian Brailean in Moose Jaw, Saskatchewan, and square dancing

In the world of dance, a serendipitous event could occur while casually reading. In Vivian's case, after her retirement and contemplating "what's next," looking at the ads in the *Moose Jaw Herald Times* newspaper was a turning point.

"I read about square dancing in the paper and thought this was a good activity," she says. "I thought that's lots of exercise, because if you dance every day and all night at a square dance, you would walk approximately five miles."

Today, Vivian is a Zone 5 representative in Moose Jaw for the Saskatchewan Square & Round Dance Federation.

## Dale and J.J. Lubberts in East Gwillimbury and social ballroom/Latin

Dale and J.J. have hardly missed any classes in their three eight-week ballroom dance sessions each year during the 2010s, run by the leisure, parks, and property department of Bradford–West Gwillimbury (pop. 35,000) in Ontario.

Travelling from their town to Bradford–West Gwillimbury because there had been no class offerings where they live, has never been an issue. Their teacher has said they are truly dedicated to dancing.

Much earlier in his life, however, J.J. says he had to repress his positive feelings about dancing because his "otherwise very good parents" approved of it only in the last few years—decades later. "I was not allowed to go to school dances … and I found out later that my mother [had] longed to go dancing."

J.J.'s actual entry into social dancing came some thirty years after he emigrated to Canada from Holland. He and Dale began dancing in the early 2000s when they both signed up for a dance class.

His later diagnosis with Parkinson's has only motivated him to continue.

"Dancing makes me feel better psychologically," says J.J. Although dancing does not directly improve his health, it has helped him enjoy the emotional benefit of dancing to music.

## Dianne and Dominic Panacci in King, Ontario, and social ballroom/Latin

Following Dominic's retirement after forty years in the conference services department at Ontario's Humber College, he added social ballroom dance classes to his walking and gym program to boost his health.

With Dianne's (his wife's) encouragement, the King Township retiree found the new experience "to do things together" fitted the bill for also advancing a closer personal connection with her.

"I was pretty active as it is, but I found dancing to be like yoga and zumba ... it was a good workout," says Dominic. "The dancing was fun and the instructor was very passionate about wanting to do things the right way ... like when you hold the partner, your right hand has to be under the shoulder blade."

## Nina Chandarana in Toronto and salsa

While at university in the late 1990s, Nina met Anuj, her husband-to-be. He was also a student and a salsa dancer. He invited her out to a salsa dance club, "where all the guys were told that if they joined the salsa club, then that's going to be their way to get girls," she recalls. On that date, "He twirled me and dipped me in the dance at one point," and those moves sealed her fate: she loved it and has never looked back. Today, after raising their children, she is a part-time salsa dance instructor at the Toronto Dance Salsa studio in North York.

## Patricia Lam in Toronto and Argentine tango

Social dancers are curious about the nature of other dance forms beyond what they have been engaged in for years. Sometimes they follow up on that curiosity. Patricia Lam was one of those. As a semi-retired older person, she began doing kizomba, salsa, and bachata after she started dancing a decade ago.

"I wanted to explore other types of dancing," she says. "A friend of mine who loves Argentine tango suggested I try it." So, she did.

## Minoo Asgary and Omar Kazi in Toronto and Argentine tango

As a budding chemical engineer in Montréal's McGill University in 1999, Omar turned to ballroom dancing on a lark one sunny summer day.

That is how he started in his now lifelong pursuit of what he today describes as an "artistic, yet creative, that's physical, yet social—activity that gives you back so much."

Minoo's pathway to her dancing was much more circuitous. As a former resident of Iran, she could only view dancing as a pipe dream due to that country's laws. In 2015, as she tried to find a dance studio near her former home in Newmarket in Ontario, she found CDA Dance Academy. But it closed its doors to adult dancing soon after she registered.

Moving to Toronto, she researched three dance studios in Toronto as part of her plan to give herself a "birthday present."

With her partner, Omar, she is now pursuing a post-working-hours agenda, focusing, since 2017, on Argentine tango, salsa, bachata, rumba, and "a little bit of ballroom."

## Pat Mastrandrea in Newmarket, Ontario, and social ballroom/Latin

Pat cut his teeth on social dancing one night by joining a long line of strangers on a Brampton, Ontario, club dance floor. "That was the one that got me up there to meet people," he says, recalling the line dance that heralded his dance leisure program for the following twenty-five years.

He enjoyed the line dancing immensely—the choreography with others who singly faced the same direction while repeating several dance figures.

His next set of moves came soon after.

At the same venue, Mastrandrea picked up another popular country dance—the two-step—this time with him holding a partner. "Two-stepping, I liked it ... I loved it," he recalls, beaming with enthusiasm.

A couple of decades later, in Newmarket where he now lives, he is still grateful for the husband-and-wife instructor couple who helped him learn the basic steps of the two-step, and the experiences he had with them are seared indelibly on his mind.

Today, he is an avid social ballroom dancer who frequents twice-monthly dances hosted by the Newmarket Seniors' Meeting Place, a facility owned by the municipality.

"I look at dance, believe it or not, as a tool that helps me in my life. That's how I look at it," he adds. "You know, we all have a variety of tools, but for me, dancing is a tool that's going to help me in my life."

## Hindy Borstein in Richmond Hill, Ontario, and "Olde Tyme" square dancing

Hindy's connection with square dancing occurred at a time when she was in her early teens and attending middle school in the north Toronto suburb of Willowdale.

She did a whole week of it during "gymnastics month" and enjoyed it thoroughly while still finding the time to learn the rules of basketball and volleyball.

The young Hindy, however, realized she was hooked on square dancing and began searching the city for it.

"After junior high, I tried finding square dancing," she says. For Hindy, it was a holy grail of sorts. When she finally located one in Harbourfront, a waterfront cultural hub in Toronto, she was disappointed it was only open to seniors.

Later, with her boyfriend, they found out about an English country dance workshop and met dancers who liked doing traditional square dancing, the "olde tyme" kind.

(Unlike modern or Western square dancing, old-time or "olde tyme" square dancing is more social in the sense that its participants learn some sets of steps and no beyond-the-basics techniques are ignored.)

"We got drawn in right away. We got hooked. That's how I finally found square dancing," she said.

## Nina Chandarana in Toronto and salsa

Currently a part-time salsa dance instructor while learning teaching skills at the Toronto Dance Salsa studio in North York, Nina says she is practising the practical concepts she has learned from her instructor such as being "grounded in your life" or connecting the dancing "to all areas of your life."

Her instructor, Aleksander Saiyan, often recommends the use of analogies (such as "you're swimming in a pool and pushing through waves") as a teaching tool. She adapts these analogies to her own classes because they make complex dance moves easier for the students to understand.

## Santha and Ivan Leong in Toronto and social ballroom/Latin

Call it a portending a union of dance minds or a marriage for life!

Ivan Leong and his future wife Santha took a few dance classes in the same space at the same place—an Arthur Murray dance studio in the Greater Toronto Area—about a year apart.

Ivan, who had not danced formally before registering as a student, got into it "because I wanted to learn something different." As well, being divorced and single for twelve years, he wanted to meet a special person in his life. His dance instructor friend, Glen Michaels, suggested he take up social dancing at his studio. Ivan later met Santha on the dancing floor, and as things turned out, Santha and Ivan later got married.

Santha got into social dancing when she was younger. She always loved social dancing, but "my parents didn't want to spend the money, so I never got to go," she says decades later. "But I got into social dancing at the Waterloo University in Ontario".

"I went with some friends and roommates. And then, after graduating from university, I started working. One day my brother said he wanted to learn dancing. So he brought me to an Arthur Murray studio that used to be next door to where he worked."

## Liboire (a.k.a. Lee) Brossard in Montréal and salsa

Lee recalls his first experience with social dancing while attending a seasonal ball hosted by a giant pharmaceutical company in Toronto. He says he did not fare well doing social ballroom dances at the event. Later, in Montréal, where he now lives, the seventy-year-old picked up—and really began to love—salsa dancing after years of physical inactivity. "I was a workaholic then," he confesses. Latin Groove studio in downtown Montréal was offering a free introductory class five nights a week, and Lee decided to attend, although at the time "I was a guy that had two left feet."

## Cristina Chirca in Montréal and salsa

Between the ages of four and fourteen, Cristina has been dancing—not salsa, but ballroom dancing. That was in Eastern Europe, where she lived until she moved to Canada. Today, she is a salsa instructor at Latin Groove in downtown Montreal.

"I started taking salsa classes—workshops, group classes … and I just fell in love with salsa," says Cristina.

## Vahide Morina in Halifax, Nova Scotia and salsa

Like most people who want to engage in dancing to balance their lifestyles, Vahide was unsure about the subtle differences between various social dance forms. As a friend of a friend suggested, she went to a salsa dance studio to check out what it was like.

She enjoyed what she saw and did. From there, she visited non-salsa studios to get a feel for other rhythms until she finally decided salsa was the dance she wanted to dedicate her spare time to.

## Marg and Larry Clark in Halifax and Argentine tango

Marg and Larry are former social ballroom dancers. In fact, they have been dancing fox trot, waltz and rumba for 53 years and during that time, they found time to teach others. In 2017, they decided to take up Argentine tango as Larry felt his knees had started to give way. The push to do so came when a family friend invited them to observe a class.

"In tango dancing, every movement and figure are like smooth 'walks'—there is no 'rise and fall' like in the waltz and fox trot," Larry explains. "It was so easy on the joints."

## Carla Anglehart in Halifax and Argentine tango

Carla came almost full circle in her dancing hobby when she "discovered," as she puts it, Argentine tango. Starting with ballet as an older child, the sixtysomething dancer has done the multiple dance forms in social ballroom and moved on to enjoy the club Latin dances such as salsa and bachata.

In 2017, however, she "fell absolutely in love with tango because of its technicality and also its improvisational nature," she says with delight. "Then there's this beautiful history to the dance … a beautiful connection you establish with the partner."

Carla's commitment to the dance has increased due to the small and dedicated tango community in Nova Scotia. "Lovely people," she remarks. "It's really the full package for me."

## Alexander Carleton in Fredericton, New Brunswick and swing

Despite a heavy academic workload for his master's degree in Calgary in the early 2010s, Alexander Carleton started dance classes to bring balance into his life.

He took up West Coast swing dancing because he was "consistent" at it. "The way it would usually work is we would have … one to two hours of dance classes on Monday nights in between [school] classes," Carleton remembers. "We had fifteen minutes of pre-dancing and then social dancing."

He later returned to Fredericton, his hometown. These days, he is a law student at the University of New Brunswick and is repeating the lifestyle pattern he set in Calgary: he is actively on the dance floor, learning Lindy Hop, a partner dance that originated in Harlem, while handling the hundreds of inquiries from potential members of the Fredericton Swing Dance (FSD) group as its public relations officer.

Alex believes he has forgotten some of his West Coast swing figures but tries his best to replicate them at social dance nights. He adds, "I like Lindy Hop because it's a kind of a goofy dance style … and I'm a goofy person."

## Kathryn Stone in Halifax, Nova Scotia and Argentine tango

Kathryn's journey into the tango started by accident. She attended a milonga to familiarize herself with what is involved. "I've always been interested in this type of tango, so I went with a male friend and I was automatically so impressed with the ways that people could move without any choreography," says Kathryn.

Observing the leg flicks by the women dancers, her friend jokingly remarked, "do their ankles just flirt?" Kathryn's rejoinder was, "Oh my gosh! I think they do."

From then on, she was hooked. "It was pretty memorable to go for the first time."

# Instructors' Guidance on the Ground

## Louise McKay and Tadahiro Okazawa in Calgary and Argentine tango

Louise says, "We are fortunate to have Leo Sato [in Calgary] as a teacher because he is very good at choreographing dance.

"I am in the social dance group, but he [Leo] also has some of the younger dancers do competitive routines involving lifts and more difficult routines. Anyway, when I started tango, I had no idea I would be able to all the things I do now—it's happening!"

## Karen Paton-Evans and Jim Evans in Shakespeare, Ontario, and social ballroom/Latin

Good social dance teachers are plentiful. But great social dancing teachers who are enthralled with teaching are rare.

Not too long ago, the Evans, who live near Woodstock, Ontario, stumbled upon the latter type of instructor as they started on their ballroom dance journey in 2007.

Referring to the Vallerands (Melody and François), who instruct in the area, Karen and Jim are excited with "… how accommodating and encouraging they are to everyone in the class.

"They put everyone at ease. We laugh a lot. Yeah, laugh a lot. You know, we laugh at ourselves," Karen says.

As for dance figures, the central parts of the dance, the Shakespeare, Ontario couple says, "Melody's choreography is always terrific—she comes up with very nice things, very interesting things."

The teacher's guidance has "greatly added to and really boosted our confidence … so now at wedding receptions [to which they are invited a lot, since Jim is a pastor], we're very comfortable on the dance floor."

As for Jim, who claims he is "introverted," he has become a "man in demand at wedding receptions, because … there will be a lineup of women of all ages waiting to dance with him one after another," says Karen. "I'm not joking."

## Jacinta Willems in Mitchell, Ontario, and Argentine tango

Starting classes at Toronto's Rhythm & Motion dance studio, Jacinta, a naturopathic doctor, has found the elements of her professional training similar to what she found in the studio. "There's a structure that is very methodical," she says. The environment is "very approachable and disciplined ... that we're going somewhere. It's not ... random. We're going in a direction and it's clear where we're going," she adds.

"I'm a disciplined person. So that's why it speaks to me, and also there is the joy that comes from the community of people in the studio that has been created," she says. "There's just a synergy in the space, and it is just super high quality, high vibrancy."

## John Loomis in Mississauga and Argentine tango

Musician, composer, and conductor John Loomis started taking Argentine tango classes several months before the pandemic arrived. With Elizabeth Sadowska of Rhythm & Motion dance studio in Toronto as his guide, he has been learning what the popular phrase "It takes two to tango" means—taking responsibility to lead the partner in the tango, a dance he has come to admire and like.

He has since been practicing his moves one hour at a time in the "tiny kitchen" at his Mississauga home.

John started attending the Saturday afternoon parties to try out his figures. "I'm still so nervous doing my steps, but what a thrill ... the lovely ladies that I practise with are very encouraging," John explains. "They help me, they coach me, and they are full of compliments."

## Andria W. in Toronto and social ballroom/Latin

When dancing socially at the 30-Up Club and the West-Way Club in Toronto, Andria is most comfortable with partners who keep the number of full spins to a minimum in a set. That is because of her vertigo, which could be momentary or long-lasting.

Otherwise, she greatly loves her dancing, as well as the instruction available at the wide range of dance studios in the Greater Toronto Area. Andria has invested in accessories that serious dancers have. "I'm the proud owner of ten dance dresses and beautiful shoes."

However, when she steps out in search of dance instruction, she is wary of "big dance schools." Recalling her first brush with the franchised "business model" of schools twenty years ago, Andria talks about the "little bit at a time [they teach you] that keeps you coming back and keeps you paying [dance instruction fees]."

It is a much different story today. At the Dance Art Studio in Richmond Hill, she showers praise on the owner and instructor, Cristina Amalia Dina, who is "not stingy with her knowledge."

Her instructor is "just all about sharing the knowledge and the love of the dance."

In the meantime, she has been dancing—except during the pandemic period—"with a lot of different people, lots of different styles, and when it's going well, it's phenomenal."

## Minoo Asgary and Omar Kazi in Toronto and Argentine tango

Since their dance partnership started, Minoo and Omar have spent a great deal of time attending group classes, semi-private classes, and even private classes, which, for many, cost a pretty penny.

Like most dancers, they dance for different reasons: one is "we do it to escape from the pressure at work," says Omar.

After reviewing the offerings of three Toronto dance studios, Minoo chose Egor Beleshov's Dance With Me Toronto studio because "Egor was very honest and very passionate about dance. [That's] what I didn't get from [the] other dance studios."

Says Omar, "We enjoy Egor's style of teaching. It's methodical—and it's good to learn about dancing from his dance stories. His method is he starts out easy, and then as we get better and better, he challenges us.

"As we practise more and more, we get more proficient so we can retain the complexity of a full sequence of steps far easier.

"We like our Argentine tango instructor a lot," adds Omar. "We have time with one another. [Egor helps me] so the experience almost became like being in a dance family. Another thing he has taught us is to be patient and learn every lesson very well."

## Cindy Stradling and Lino in Toronto and social ballroom/Latin

Long before Cindy met her boyfriend, Lino, she used to spend time attending public events. One evening at a social get-together in the 1990s, she accepted a dance request.

"That's the first time I started dancing, and [my partner] was a really good dancer," Cindy recalls. "I learned a lot from him … and that sort of planted the seed" in pursuing dancing in a more choreographed way.

Seven years ago, she met Lino, to whom she was introduced by a friend. Together, they have been learning the American style of social ballroom dancing and have picked up some cool moves in the cha-cha-cha, rumba, waltz, and salsa.

Before the pandemic, "we went out at least once or twice a month," says Cindy. "Sometimes on a Saturday night, we'd put on some music and do just a little bit of practicing."

Since Cindy's first dance, she and Lino have grown a lot. "We both said this is what we want to do. We both want to be able to know what to do, what [dance] steps to take, because it's easy to do the old free-flow dancing [the way people without studio training dance]," says Cindy.

At some Toronto dance venues they have visited, including the Capitol, the 30-Up, and the Old Mill, they try their best to remember the social ballroom steps learned in the past and use them.

"With the cha-cha-cha steps, you can do a lot," she says.

## Liboire (a.k.a. Lee) Brossard in Montréal and salsa

Lee counts himself as one of the luckiest salsa dancers in Canada. Regarding Sandra Campanelli, the owner of Latin Groove (where he first started salsa dancing in 2007, considered one of the top three dance studios in Montréal in 2020), he says she is gifted and talented, as well as passionate about salsa. "She has a unique way of explaining things—footwork, body movement, and everything else," Lee explains.

"Her studio is also about creating a community atmosphere through dancing and events—balls, parties—bringing people together," he says. "That's what really kept me plugged in."

# Practising the Moves

## Diane Ternan and David Franks in Newmarket, Ontario and social ballroom/Latin

"When we're practising at home, we sometimes have a different memory of how the steps go and also don't remember what were taught and agree on what we were taught.

"We tried a couple of times doing it like the video, looking at the YouTube videos. But … watching those videos and how they do it can be confusing because they may be doing American style, and we do the International-style [in ballroom]."

"Then, after a few tries at something, we really can't get it. Sometimes we just agree to leave that piece alone until we get back to class."

## Santha and Ivan Leong in Markham, Ontario and social ballroom/Latin

Says Santha, "We don't have a place where there's enough space. So, much of our dance practice we do in our small space at home."

She notes that "Ivan finds it challenging to learn new steps and so finds dancing very stressful."

Ivan, on the other hand, says Santha is always excited to attend classes and practice. "She loves dancing ten thousand times more than I do. She is a much better dancer than I am by a long way. She automatically goes into it and does well. For me, it's not as natural—I have to work very hard at it."

Ivan adds, "I learn by way of patterns, and then I memorize a pattern to do a dance step."

## Monika Szymczak in Toronto and social ballroom/Latin

In her job as an Ontario correctional officer, Monika has been highly trained to be alert and prepared to react to the unexpected. Practicing with a partner one evening at a Toronto ballroom dance club, she recalls the lead changing the structure of figures she knew well.

"It's still important to follow his lead; you have to follow him even if he may not be doing [them] perfectly … just follow him," says Monika. "That way, you'll be more adjustable and flexible for him [and] he will not struggle with you, although you know he's doing it wrong. It doesn't matter if someone is doing it right or wrong."

## Patricia Lam in Toronto and Argentine tango

Patricia had decided, two years ago, to devote herself exclusively to Argentine tango, although she previously enjoyed dancing bachata, kizomba, and salsa. After viewing a Stardust Dance Productions performance of tango in New York a while ago, she realized "how beautiful this dance is," and "it seems to instil a sense of discipline that one has to take seriously."

Joining the Bulent and Tina dance studio in Toronto, she was impressed by the manner in which one of the principal instructors "helped me in my transition into the tango." Patricia says the instructor "was always encouraging and patient with me, despite how busy she was during the lesson."

## Jacinta Willems in Mitchell, Ontario and Argentine tango

Jacinta started learning the tango half a year before the pandemic began. She knew early she did not want "to dabble" in her newfound interest, so she set out to find an "excellent" teacher. Connecting with instructor Elizabeth Sadowska in Toronto, Jacinta has been travelling 350 km. to take lessons, along with the afternoon practice sessions, making it a full-day event.

In addition to her formal training time, she has organized space in her home so she can do her moves in front of a mirror. She practices four times a week. The call to "practice, practice, practice" has become "a huge motivator" because she knows how good preparation will help deal with "my hunger to learn the dance well enough so that when I am participating in social dancing, the magic will happen," she says.

## Pat Mastrandrea in Newmarket, Ontario, and social ballroom/Latin

"How do I start this 'thing?'" is the question Pat poses to himself when he does not remember his dance steps.

"Once I get that under my belt, it comes out pretty good," says Pat.

He recalls telling his dance partner during the second wave of the coronavirus pandemic that "if [it] carries on for four months, geez, we're going to forget all our dance steps.

"So we've got to practise in 2021, down in the basement."

## Cindy Stradling in Toronto and social ballroom/Latin

The biggest challenges for Cindy and her dance partner are "getting the step right" and making missteps due to being distracted.

According to her, when they are dancing socially, they may look at another couple and get derailed from what they are doing,

Her partner needs to be a stronger lead, she says. Once they achieve that, they can rely on their instructor, Cristina Amalia Dana at the Dance Art Studio, to learn how to better memorize dance figures and to prevent themselves from being distracted, especially when dancing in public.

## Andria W. in Toronto and social ballroom/Latin

Social dancers often resort to visualization techniques to retain knowledge they have learned in their dance classes. Andria is one of them.

"I think about them [the steps]. Sometimes I lie in bed at night waiting to fall asleep, thinking about them," she explains. "I really hope I don't forget it all and have to start from scratch."

## Vahide Morina in Halifax and salsa

Being a personal trainer, Vahide understands how instructions, advice, and personal examples can motivate her clients to be successful. As a salsa student in Trena's Studio, she has seen those skills practised by her instructor, Trena Graham.

"She knows what to say to you that works for your body," says Vahide. "With some figures, I may get overwhelmed … so she'd say 'just focus on this part and then this part'—that helps a lot.

"Trena certainly looks at each student as an individual and uses tools to help them understand the dance," she explains.

## Alexander Carleton in Fredericton, New Brunswick and swing

Alexander started dancing with West Coast swing in Calgary. Returning to New Brunswick, the Fredericton native is learning Lindy Hop at the Fredericton's Swing Dance) club.

"I feel miserable when I feel I've forgotten something, and with COVID I feel like I've forgotten everything. But I'm a little more comfortable now [during the second wave of the pandemic].

"When I forget something, I ask someone to work through it with me, like just saying, 'Hey, do you remember this?' or ask someone you know, and with their permission, try to get it."

## Cristina Chirca in Montréal and salsa

Cristina, a Latin Groove dance studio instructor, knows well how to get the best out of the dancers under her charge.

Her experiences as a student have taught her a lot about creating the ideal environment for practicing salsa. She recalls her student days in Montréal, where "the environment was so welcoming and friendly that you felt you wanted to be there at all times."

"If you were falling behind, nobody was there to point fingers," she explains. "Everybody helped out one another, and the teachers were very helpful."

# Most Enjoyable Moments Dancing

## Timothy Tan in Vancouver and social ballroom/Latin

A favourite moment for Vancouver's Timothy Tan was at a recent social dance that he and his partner attended before the pandemic struck.

Tan, a former president of the University of British Columbia Dance Club, says they were both familiar with a choreographed routine, and they happened on "just the right" piece of music.

"It was about the song first and foremost. We felt a good chemistry, a good vibe, and the dancing became less of a structural mechanical process.

"It was a relationship [between us] expressed publicly on a dance floor and there was an explosive joy to it," he recalls.

## Arkady Silverman in Toronto and social ballroom/Latin

A dedicated, long-time student of Mandy's Dance studio in Mississauga, Arkady also has spent hundreds of hours watching YouTube dancing videos to complement her knowledge.

Her most significant experience on the dance floor was in the 2010s in western England during the annual Blackpool Junior Dance Festival, which is usually held in late spring. She took a stab at competing in the student competition.

"I would come home [where I was staying]. Mandy and I would develop my choreography, and then I would take the routine back with me to my partner to compete with," recalls twentysomething Arkady.

"It was an outstanding experience and really satisfied my childhood expectations after watching Blackpool videos from a young age," she says.

## Alice Meinecke in Bracebridge, Ontario, and square dancing

A square-dancing aficionado, Alice speaks as an enthusiastic follower of this genre of dancing: "We're a dancing community [where] it's great exercise, great music, and it's real fun."

"No one at the square dance can be unhappy." With snappy country music in the background, the Bracebridge woman is totally in the moment on the dance floor. "I'm thinking about the caller and I'm listening to the rhythm of the music.

"I'm moving through the dance as the caller is instructing me to do. I'm really moving to the music, feeling the music … and that is pretty good."

Alice usually has a great time as she dances in her square!

## Sandra Holliday-Tucker and Silas ("Sie") Tucker in Newmarket and social ballroom/Latin

According to Sie, the high point in his dancing with Sandra is "when we could actually go around the entire dance floor [in a counter-clockwise direction] without bumping into somebody and actually doing the moves that I want to do.

"It doesn't happen all the time because you're either running into people or forgetting a particular move," he says.

"So, when I can go around the dance floor with Sandra, I feel that I've done a really good job, and it's very enriching for me," Sie says gleefully. "It makes me very happy."

Adds Sandra, "When it works well, it feels almost as though you're just flowing; everything flows."

## Nina Chandarana in Toronto and salsa

Nina's recollection of a most enjoyable time out dancing was with Anuj, her husband, who was her first salsa partner more than two decades ago. One evening, with the kids being looked after by her parents, she and Anuj attended a salsa dance. "It was a really beautiful event!" she says. Nina was able to introduce her husband to her dance friends.

When Anuj and Nina, "There was something beyond the physical connection of dancing. There was that emotional, deep connection I felt—just like in the Cuban motion connection.

"It was a reminder that we do fit like a glove. Beautiful!"

## Monika Szymczak in Toronto and social ballroom/Latin

Recalling her most memorable experience with a partner at a dance, Monika says, "As I dance, I'm just going with the flow, listening to the music. And just feel like I am so light. Like, you know, almost not feeling my weight, and then just the mood, the mood, the music moves me.

"And if I know bigger steps, then of course it's the best expression with the partner. Then I know how to respond to his leading, because I know the steps. That's the biggest pleasure!"

## Karen Paton-Evans and Jim Evans in Shakespeare, Ontario, and social ballroom/Latin

When chatting about a high point in dancing, some couples call it "a magic moment." Karen and Jim's special term for it is "a sweet spot."

"That move that we've been trying so hard to happen, happens," Karen explains. "Now all of a sudden, it clicks … it works."

In a dance class practice, "When other dancers see us do a routine or figure that is challenging, they're just as thrilled as we are … they are happy for us."

## Patricia Lam in Toronto and Argentine tango

In 2019, not too long after Patricia began her tango dancing, she attended a *milonga* where she danced with a partner who had been practicing tango for more than twenty-five years.

"I felt transported into a 'Zen' trance," she recalls.

Today, there is no looking back. With the limited time she has available for dancing, the focus is on "one dance," in contrast with her earlier decade of doing bachata, kizomba, and salsa concurrently.

## Liboire (a.k.a. Lee) Brossard in Montréal and salsa

Lee says he appreciates the session parties that Latin Groove studio offers every six weeks. "It's a highlight because there is a golden rule: Nobody could say no to a person asking for a dance, whether you're a beginner or at a higher level." Those parties, for him, are a big deal, since he likes dressing up.

"You know what? I've got seven pairs of dance shoes!"

At these sessions, he dances "three to four hours non-stop with different ladies I know," he says. "And just letting go and just being there in the moment with the music with my different partners."

He usually gets home exhausted and collapses into bed. The best feeling for him, however, is on the following morning, "I have the biggest smile on my face."

## Vahide Morina in Halifax, Nova Scotia and salsa

Vahide started learning salsa in March, a year before the COVID-19 pandemic, and for that year before the shutdown of dance studios, she danced a lot. The high for her in salsa dancing comes when she and her partner hit the same beat perfectly or "I or the other person do a move or something, and you feed off the other person and respond with something really similar—that I think was probably the most enjoyable," she says. "It's so unexpected, and for you to be still connected … it almost feels magical."

## Marg and Larry Clark in Halifax and Argentine tango

One of Marg's better memories doing the so-called "Dance of Embraces" with Larry was at a formal *milonga* where people are dressed to the nines. "We were standing on the floor and doing what we've been taught to do without breaking up," recalls Marg. "You just have to go with the flow … no stopping … and if one of you makes a mistake, you just carry on as if nothing happened."

## Carla Anglehart in Halifax and Argentine tango

It was the summer of 2020 when Carla experienced the most enjoyable time doing the tango. Although the pandemic was raging everywhere, Carla with her mask on, danced many evenings away with her dance partner at the Halifax waterfront.

The ambience each evening was right: cool breezes blowing in from the ocean, the smell of cooking, tango music in the background, and "being able to sort of just allow yourself to express yourself through the dance and being in tune with him [my partner]."

"With COVID, "we haven't been able to sort of go out and do things that are special as much as we would in the past," Carla adds. "So when I knew that what we were doing along the waterfront was so nice and having to get dressed with a flowing dress and feel like, you know, feel beautiful and then have the experience of all of those great sensations and what not. It was really lovely.

"I felt like I was in heaven."

## Vaunda and Martin Vanderaa in Charlottetown, Prince Edward Island and square dancing

The most memorable moments for Vaunda and Martin in square dancing came in 2019. They drove to Fredericton, New Brunswick, from their Charlottetown home to attend the annual "mecca" held for the Atlantic provinces' square dancers. It was a whole weekend affair. "We loved the exercise and the friendship" of the various dancers. "The callers were in tune and played the right music and the right beat."

# Conclusion

There is, perhaps, no doubt that the voices of dancers expressed here represent the wide range of emotions and general feelings experienced by Canadians when they dance in private balls, clubs, public dance halls and pavilions, hotel dining rooms, bars, and in their home kitchens and family rooms.

Research suggests that Canadians pursue some 190 forms of dance for social and professional reasons.[4]

To dance, whether professionally or socially, is to enter a different world: a world of sheer joyousness, pleasure, and exercise. Some have suggested that dance is their therapy.

One thing is certain: history shows, as also noted in the first chapter of the book, that Canadians love to dance. They have found solace in dance as a means of getting away temporarily from the daily grind of working. This is still true today.

The persons interviewed in this chapter, however, have expressed or implied that during the 2020–2021 pandemic, they have been starved of dance classes and barred from public dance places. Like millions of others engaged in other leisure pursuits, their mental health has suffered, hopefully not irreparably.

Some have taken to the streets to protest. In the afternoon of March 1, 2021, a 15-year-old Barrie, Ontario dance student led a three-hour protest at the City of Barrie Hall, claiming unfairness in a decision regarding COVID-19 restrictions by the Simcoe Muskoka District Health Unit.

"Simcoe County Schools are running large classes of dance students where students are eating and yet dance studios that take temperatures, sanitize, have half as many students in a room and do not allow food are being shut down," said Lexi Cooper.[5]

Governmental restrictions that started in March 2020 are continuing with the "third wave" of the virus occurring during the first six months of 2021.

(There has been speculation of a possible "fourth wave" at the time of writing.)

---

[1] Chris Thorburn. www.kelownaballroom.com/about.html, accessed 10 October 2020.

[2] Lewis Carroll and John Tenniel. *Alice's Adventures in Wonderland,* London: SDE Classics, 2019.

[3] Square and Round Dancers of South Western Ontario. https://swosda.ca/ accessed 6 January 2021

[4] Canada Council for the Arts. *Yes, I dance: A survey of who dances in Canada.* Ottawa: accessed 21 July 2014

[5] Janis Ramsay, "Dance studios holding rolling protests at Barrie city hall," *Barrie Advance*, 28 February 2021, Dance studios holding rolling protest at Barrie City Hall (simcoe.com) accessed 2 April 2021

# Chapter 3: Joyful Moments for Special Dancers

The best time in Halifax every year, residents say, is spring. That is when the bushes and flowerbeds in its historic public gardens in the middle of the city come to life after the winter. For Nova Scotia's adults with Parkinson's disease, the spring of 2013 could not have come earlier; it symbolized another season of hope for better things.

On a beautiful Saturday afternoon that season, Tea & Tango, an Argentine tango dance class designed for persons with neurological conditions, started in the provincial capital. It was the brainchild of instructor duo Martina Sommer and Lorne Buick.

The launch event was attended by observers that included occupational therapists and physiotherapists. "I saw people with PD began moving in different directions … because of being engaged with the music," Sommer recalls.

It was clearly a "complete experience," recalls Sommer, who, along with Buick, also runs the downtown You, Two, Can Tango dance studio. "It wasn't just the joy of dancing but also the socializing with others facing similar circumstances. It was unbelievable happening," she says. "The whole class was filled with laughter and smiling faces. It was very humbling, I have to say."

Following the launch, Sommer told a CBC News reporter that it was important that "everyone has a chance to dance because dancing is one of the most important aspects of human life—we have just forgotten about it."[1]

Since that first dance party in 2013, Tea & Tango has been running as a weekly social dance event, thanks to a long parade of helpers, including its first volunteers, graphic designer Julia Zalvalna and Jesse Robson, founder of the seniors' charity Happily Ever Active.

# Wheelchair-Bound Dancers

With a one-time grant from Arts Nova Scotia in 2013, Tea & Tango was also able to introduce wheelchair dancing for five persons and their able-bodied partners or volunteers. This was Nova Scotia's first social dance event to help reduce the isolation of wheelchair-bound persons with various disabilities, including Parkinson's disease (PD).

"Those who participated were connected, with their arms, to another person," Sommer explains. "It was astonishing how much movement there was on bodies that were on wheelchairs."

The first dance school in Canada to offer classes for students on wheelchairs was the Chance Dance Centre in Ontario, according to Sergey Muretov, the studio owner. He ran similar classes in Ukraine before immigrating to Canada.

With studios in both Newmarket and Georgina, towns north of Toronto, Muretov says his studio "wants to make sure that all people are able to experience the joy of dance [2]... Dancing is dancing, whether you are standing or sitting," is his motto. "Rhythm and music are from inside the body and the mind."[3]

In 2013, Wheel Dance, a Toronto non-profit, has been providing wheelchair ballroom and Latin dance classes to individuals "with ambulatory disabilities along with able-bodied individuals."[4] The organization received financial assistance from the Ontario Trillium Foundation, a provincial community-building fund.

Louise Russo, an affiliate of the Toronto-based Gluckstein Personal Injury Lawyers and Wheel Dance, is quoted on the law firm's website, explaining that wheelchair dancing "...promotes physical, social and psychological benefits, plus it enables and supports the integration of disabled individuals into the community."

Russo added, "Rehab professionals are supportive, involved, and excited to be promoting it." She is co-chair of the Canadian Coalition for Mobility Challenged Drivers.

As early as 2008, other dance programs rolled out to help banish the isolation felt by people with PD, using dancing to mitigate symptoms and the impacts on their health.

In 2008, for instance, Toronto-based Sarah Robichaud started Dancing with Parkinson's (DWP) and offered—and still offers—dance classes in more than fifteen locations throughout the Greater Toronto Area. Using the training she received in New York's Mark Morris Dance Company, she has inspired hundreds of persons with Parkinson's disease to dance and reap the benefits, including better body balance, motor skills, and physical confidence.

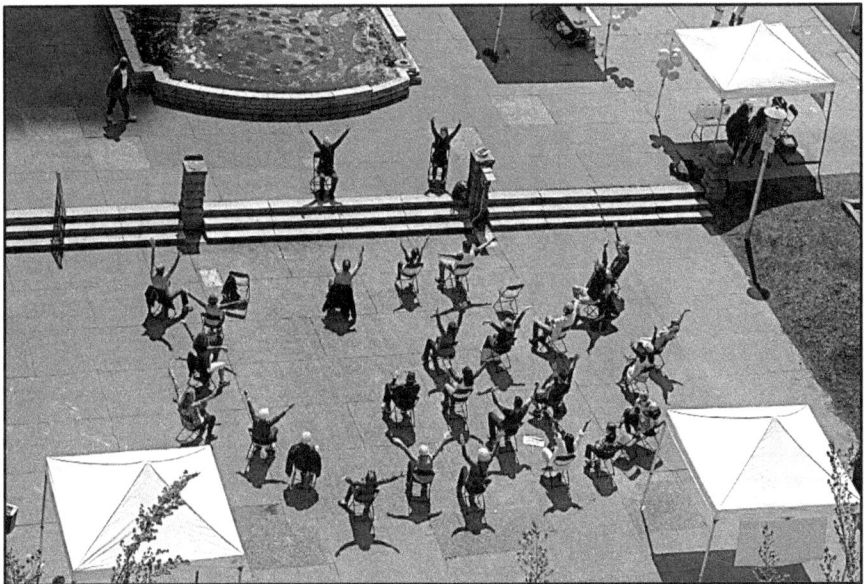

Figure 7

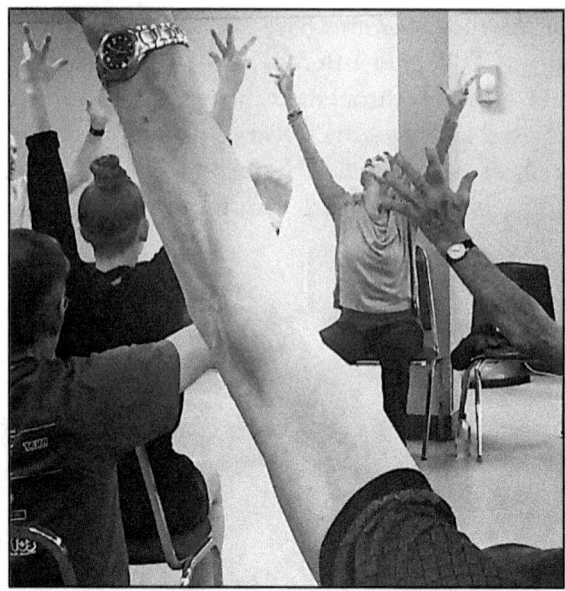

Figure 7 and 8: Indoor participants from the U.S., Central Canada and B.C. celebrate with dance movements using extended arms at the RISE exercise and wellness retreat for individuals with Parkinson's, at Trinity Western University in Langley, B.C. Outdoor event was o organized in June 2018 by NeuroFit BC.

# Organizations Pitch In

With a growing and aging population, it is estimated that the number of Canadians living with parkinsonism will double between 2011 and 2031 and that the incidence will increase by 50%.[5] (Parkinsonism is an umbrella term that includes Parkinson's disease, secondary parkinsonism, and atypical parkinsonism.)

Parkinson's disease is a chronic degenerative disorder of the central nervous system. Brain cells that control muscle movement are destroyed, and this results in symptoms that include tremors, loss of balance, stiff limbs, and frequent falls.

Support by various organizations to help persons with PD has scaled up considerably over the years. Dance for Parkinson's Network Canada (DFPNC) is an umbrella organization that was established to take on the challenge. It is a partnership of Canada's National Ballet School (NBS)/Sharing Dance, Dancing with Parkinson's, and Parkinson Canada, and Dance for PD.

Karen Lee, CEO of Parkinson Canada in Toronto, says her organization's earlier funding of research into Parkinson's disease helped the NBS's Sharing Dance project come to fruition.

During one of the government-ordered lockdowns during the COVID-19 pandemic, the famous ballet school with its twelve dance studios located in the Celia Franca Centre building in Toronto hosted virtual classes for its Sharing Dance Parkinson's community program students. Classes began with seated dancing, followed by dancing in a standing position. The sessions were flexible; those who preferred to dance in a seated position throughout the session were allowed.

Dance for PD, a community program of the Mark Morris Dance Group in New York, has been running dozens of classes for people with Parkinson's disease, as well as for their families, friends, and care partners. Classes are held in church halls and community halls from British Columbia to Newfoundland and Labrador.

Like other Dance for PD groups, the PD project, officially called Dance Class for People Living with Parkinson's, in Saskatoon, Saskatchewan, owes its success to volunteers and caregivers, according to dance instructor Shannon Bray, who runs dance sessions at McClure United Church.

Partnering with the church's pastor, Parkinson's Saskatchewan, local neurologists, and community groups, Bray, assisted by her sister, Robyn, has shaped, since September of 2018, a weekly program based on the intensive training she received at Toronto's National Ballet School (NBC).

The courses she took include the Dancing for Parkinson's teacher training program and the Baycrest/NBS dance course for people with dementia.

Enrolment in the Saskatoon project has been strengthened as the church "has an attached seniors' tower and a senior's assisted living complex," Bray says. "We have some of our dance members living in those communities."

In British Columbia, dancer Megan Walter Straight has her hands full travelling between Vancouver, North Vancouver, West Vancouver, and Coquitlam with her PD classes. "I'd have probably in each class anywhere from fifteen to twenty people or maybe more—attendance varies," Straight says.

She sees her mission as one that "provides help to people with similar challenges to find movement in their bodies and significantly to explore our sense of community together.

"There's a lot of smiling in the classes," Straight adds. The people who come "find they are in a safe place where they can explore moving their bodies, where typically they might feel uncomfortable doing that."

In her classes, Straight says, "they can refine their sense of motion and that sense of dance we all have in ourselves, and they are doing so with a physical condition that works against that."

Downtown Montreal's Belgo Building, which is widely known for housing dozens of contemporary art galleries, is also the site of dance classes for PD. Instructor Tania has been running them since 2015 and is pleased with the results. "Everything is organized in a way that the dancers may forget the disease."

In Charlottetown, Prince Edward Island, Irene Doyle, organizer of the Movers and Shakers group, runs rumba dance classes for persons with PD. At the Central Christian Church, all classes are held "sitting down," says Doyle, and led by a Zumba instructor who is a retired university professor.

# Various Dance Forms for Dancers with Disabilities

Research has shown that dancing can improve the social, physical, and mental well-being of adults with disabilities. Dance instructors who specifically devote their time to this group are part of a growing movement called dance/movement therapy (DMT). Dance teachers working with persons with PD are being increasingly recognized within healthcare and mental health circles as invaluable in rehabilitation work.

Dance instructors who operate for the Dance for PD organization use various dance forms in their work.

The Toronto-based Dancing for Parkinson's classes engage their dancers with ballet, modern, Broadway, Latin, tango, swing, and jazz.[6] Dancing with Parkinson's Megan Walter Straight in B.C. also uses a similar host of dance forms. "I use everything I can think of, including all kinds of music," says Straight.

Patricia McKinley, professor emerita at Montreal's McGill University's school of physical and occupational therapy, has specialized in researching the specific value of one particular dance, Argentine tango, for promoting health and well-being.

In a joint study with Gammon Earhart, a professor at Washington University, she found that adults who danced tango to rehabilitate from the fear of falling (after experiencing a "slip and fall" episode) gained more improvements in balance and motor coordination than those who did walking for the same purpose.

As a general exercise choice for older adults, McKinley says "tango dancing is an ideal leisure activity for this population. It satisfies three basic requirements for exercise adherence: it's fun, it's a group activity, and it has a tangible goal that can be perceived not only by the dancer, but also by his or her family and friends."[7]

Other mental health advocates, too, are recognizing dance as a remedy to suppressing PD symptoms. As recently as 2020, neuroscientists Lydia Giménez-Llort and Lidia Castillo-Mariqueo have presented evidence that *paso doble*, a Latin ballroom dance, is as effective as Argentine tango in that regard.

Both professors, who teach at Spain's Universitat Autònoma de Barcelona, have proposed that *paso doble* is a therapeutic exercise for PD while providing what they call "a protective strategy" for caregivers.

"*Paso doble* can also contribute to improving physical capacity and all its components. Besides, [it] is also a music per se, with familiarity and groove that compels to move which can serve as an external reference to facilitate specific movements," they explain.

> We consider that this easy to implement into patient care and free-living environments (elderly social centers, home) rehabilitation program can promote positive emotions and self-esteem, with added general improvement of social attachment and recognition, thus improving the quality of life of patient caregiver as a patient and family caregiving intervention that can be tailored to the individuals.[8]

## Argentine Tango, a Boon to the Life of Two Nova Scotia Dancers with PD

Colin Hill, Paul Parks, and their wives live in Halifax.

Apart from being older adults, the men also cope daily with the inconveniences of having Parkinson's disease (PD). They met each other only recently when they, along with their respective wives, Valery and Theresa, attended the weekly Tea & Tango sessions in the city a couple of years ago.

Now they have become friends and sometimes find time to play cards and visit the city's waterfront. "We feel very easy with each other because we all have similar concerns," says Colin.

Another activity they have shared while the pandemic raged on, and which they both find exciting, is writing; they have written fiction. "It's kind of socializing in a way, especially when we read each other's stories," says Paul.

As for the dancing, they both feel they are the beneficiaries in executing the sultry movements of the Argentine tango.

Remembering his first steps in 2017, Paul says after five minutes on the floor with Theresa, "I was quite surprised to feel I moved a little more freely for a few minutes. Doing the tango for as little as five minutes, my muscles became much more relaxed. I was actually quite surprised to find that out."

He says he is always "conscious of my physical limitations," but while on the dance floor, "it was so nice to embrace Theresa" in an Argentine tango hold and do the *promenade* figure.

Colin is on the same wavelength. "I'm so glad we found it, because it's been such a worthwhile thing to do for the last couple of years."

"Our learning sessions at Tea & Tango are only about an hour, then we would have a tea break followed by socializing—talking with each other about life and dancing and so forth," he says.

The wives are happy to tag along with their husbands to the weekly parties. Colin's wife, Valery, is quick to say how much she has enjoyed "following the music and the dance patterns that Martina (the instructor) has taught us.

"The sidestep and the back walk, you know, all those things—they are really terrific," she says.

Valery notes that before Colin was diagnosed with Parkinson's disease in the early 2000s, they both took ballroom dancing for five years. "We never really got into Argentine tango before the last set of classes ended."

At their respective homes, the two men say they practise the moves they learned at the tea parties for practical reasons. Theresa says they push aside the kitchen table to dance when Paul feels stressed. "I'd just say to Paul, 'You want to tango?' and then we'd put on the music for five minutes, and he'd feel better."

"Dancing has also helped Paul's posture," she says.

# Conclusion

Public health researchers emphasize the need to keep physically active. It is a goal, they say, that everyone, regardless of age, should strive toward achieving a healthier lifestyle.

Among the hundreds of physical activities available to everyone is dance. A 2014 study by the Canada Council for the Arts states that Canadians pursue 190 types of dancing, ranging from Argentine tango to Armenian dances to Afro-Caribbean, for personal enjoyment, exercise and therapy, and for work purposes.

For people with disabilities, most, if not all, can access these dance genres once there are instructors or amenities available in their communities.

One characteristic of dancing that stands out for people with special needs is that it can potentially improve health, not only physically, but also emotionally and spiritually. Furthermore, these positive benefits have been proven to link to higher self-esteem and coping strategies. Good examples of all these benefits are the brief stories of Paul Parks and Colin Hill above.

Over the past two decades, much research has been devoted specifically to the benefits of dancing among adults with Parkinson's disease. The 2015 work by the Evaluation Centre for Complex Health Interventions (TEC-CHI) at the University of Toronto may be relevant.

The classes, sponsored by the Toronto-based Dancing with Parkinson's (DWP) organization, brought participants out of isolation and into the community, where they had an opportunity to benefit emotionally and physically through dance.

The year-long evaluation, funded by the Ontario Brain Institute Evaluation Support Program, explored how DWP made a difference in the lives of people with Parkinson's disease.[9]

---

[1] CBC News. "Neurological patients learn to tango in Halifax: Social sharing: Dancers hve Alzheimer's and Parkinson's disease". https://www.cbc.ca/news/canada/nova-scotia/neurological-patients-learn-to-tango-in-halifax-1.2433114 accessed 13 March 2021.

[2] "Wheelchair dance classes", http://chancedancecentre.com/, accessed 28 March 2021

[3] Ibid.

[4] https://www.gluckstein.com/introducing-wheel-dance-wheelchair-dancesport/, accessed 27 March 2021.

[5] Public Health Agency of Canada (PHAC), Neurological health charities Canada (NHCC). *Mapping connections: An understanding of neurological conditions in Canada.* Ottawa: 2014. (cited 2017 July 12) Report no.: HP35-45/2014E-PDF, accessed 14 March 2021.

[6] "Introducing wheel dance & wheelchair dancesport" https://www.gluckstein.com/introducing-wheel-dance-wheelchair-dancesport/ accessed 27 March 2021.

[7] McGill Newsroom press release. "Shall we dance: Doing the tango improves the aging brain," Montreal: McGill University. 23 November 2005, https://www.mcgill.ca/newsroom/channels/news/shall-we-dance-1760, accessed 20 March 2021.

[8] Giménez-Llort, L. & Castillo-Mariqueo, L. " PasoDoble, a proposed dance/music for people With Parkinson's disease and their caregivers," *Frontiers in Neurology*, 12 November 2020. https://www.frontiersin.org/articles/10.3389/fneur.2020.567891/full accessed March 27 2021.

[9] "Arts and dance related evaluations: Dancing with Parkinson's," https://torontoevaluation.ca/centre/?page_id=74, accessed 3 February 2021.

# Chapter 4: The Dance Academy—Watching Over Dancers Each Step of the Way

> Beginner dancer: knows nothing. Intermediate dancer: knows everything but is too good to dance with beginners. Hotshot dancer: too good to dance with anyone. Advanced dancer: dances everything, especially with beginners.—Deniz Karakulak, principal, Toronto Dance Professionals

On a frosty December evening in 2020 during the second wave of the COVID-19 pandemic, a dozen couples stood in their own living room ready to dance with other couples across Alberta.

Joined through a Zoom video conference, each couple could at least see the other couples ready to dance with them. Once the couple formations were ready, square dance caller Barrie McCombs' voice boomed out the details of a dance figure.

Minutes later, smiling, the dance couples had all executed a warm-up "do-si-do" dance step that McCombs prompted.

This lesson was one of many virtual dance classes run by Square Dance Calgary, the moniker for the Calgary & District Square and Round Dancers Association, which includes dozens of area clubs.

As for hundreds of instructors in other dance forms such as salsa, Argentine tango and social ballroom, many of them also hosted virtual dance instruction in their studios for their students at home.

Teachers of dance had no choice but to go virtual. For some, it was an opportunity to recoup lost revenue. It is estimated that the average dance teacher in Canada experienced a loss of or faced 36 "gigs" at risk. Each independent dance teacher, along with other artists and cultural workers, lost varying levels of income, according to *I Lost My Gig*, an impact study of COVID-19 by a research firm.

In normal times, social dancers learn mainly through in-person training, through studio classes, practices, and parties. Overall, they depend on the so-called "dance academy" to look good—and also feel good—on the dance floor.

The Canadian social dance academy is an intricate web of independent dance schools, studios, recreational or community dance clubs in secondary schools, colleges and universities across the country.

It also includes YouTube videos, websites, books on dance techniques, and various dance workshops and festivals run by dance professionals.

At the heart of the academy are the instructors—social ballroom dance teachers, salsa instructors, Argentine tango experts and square dance teachers/callers, and round dance cuers. They are the front-line providers of dance knowledge and the dance step fixers.

There is even a special academy for professional dance teachers and those aspiring to be.

At one time or another, dance instructors, like other professionals, go to school to learn the dance forms that they teach social dancers. To find out how instructors get trained, the Canada Council for the Arts (the Council) undertook, in 2014, a wide-ranging study of Canadian dancing. To finalize the Canada Dance Mapping Study, the Council launched the *Yes I Dance* survey.

The survey found that six out of ten professionals turned to dance schools, studios and dance training academies for their training. Women instructors were considerably more likely than men to have learned dance through a school.[2]

Many dance instructors and instructors-in-training hire competitive dance champions as "their dance school." The champions are usually members of the Canadian DanceSport Federation (CDF), which has an eight-person panel of examiners, two of whom focus on Argentine tango, to certify their members. The federation's mission "is to foster a professional dance community from coast to coast." The federation explains,[3] "We do this through facilitating education, collaboration with each other, assisting the development of social and competitive dancesport throughout our vast country."

Another dance examining body is the Canadian Dance Teachers' Association (CDTA) which grants teacher certification in both International

Style ballroom, International Style Latin, as well as American style "smooth" and "rhythm."

# The Ballroom/Latin Academy

Dance professionals primarily teach social ballroom and other social dances in Canada, work and reside in cities and towns from British Columbia to Newfoundland. Most of them ply their professional skills in privately-owned dance studios and for-profit or volunteer-run social dance clubs. Some even have home studios that are more than double the size of an average one-bedroom apartment.

Instructors often cross over and instruct in the social ballroom dance classes run by municipal governments' leisure services departments. (More information on this option comes at the end of this chapter.)

## Seasoned Practitioners Lead the Pack

Dance champions, crackerjack dancesport competitors and CDTA-certified instructors are among the hundreds of social dance teachers in Canada. Because the social ballroom dance industry is not regulated by Canadian governments, highly experienced but uncertified teachers also teach.

Over the past few decades, thousands of social ballroom dancers from coast-to-coast have received training from these instructors.

Let's meet a few experts in the social ballroom field:

**George** and **Wendy Pytlik** of British Columbia, own Delta Dance in the Greater Vancouver Area. They are certified dance instructors and former two-time SnowBall Classic Latin champions in their age group. They also finished 27th in the 2010 Senior 1 World Championship Ten Dance competition.

**Magda Rudzik** and **Andrew McIntosh** are co-founders of Dancing for Dessert Ballroom and Latin Dance Studio in Langley, BC. Having trained in Canada and in England with the world's top dance coaches, they competed internationally and in 2004 were featured as the inaugural ballroom and Latin dance team onboard the Queen Mary 2, the British transatlantic ocean liner and the world's largest cruise ship at that time. After teaching and performing on the high seas, they opened their studio in 2005 and have since taught thousands of students the joys of partner dancing.

**Delphine Romaire** and **Dominic Lacroix** are highly trained and accomplished dancers who own Elite Dance Studio in Edmonton. They have shared titles such as former eight-time Amateur Canadian champions; 16-time Amateur Québec champions; North American Standard champions; and 19-time Canadian representatives at World Championships.

**Anna Borshch**, along with her partner **Anton Lebedev**, runs a franchised Arthur Murray dance studio in Ajax, Ontario. She is a former eight-time Canadian ballroom professional champion,

**Cristina Amalia Dina**, owner of Dance Art Studio in Richmond Hill, Ontario, is a former dancesport champion in "Ten-Dance." She is a licentiate with the Canadian Dance Teachers' Association (CDTA) an associate member of the Canadian DanceSport Federation (CDF)

**Mandy Epprecht** owns Mandy's Dance in Mississauga, Ontario. She is a former competitor on the world stage—a two-time representative to the World Professional Championships in 1990 and 1992 and represented Canada at the World Ten Dance competition in 1990. A licentiate with both the CDF and the International Dance Teachers' Association ("highly commended"), she is a 16-year Canadian professional finalist in dancesport. Epprecht is also a lifetime member of the World Salsa Federation.

**Maxim Fomin**, a former North American vice-champion and Québec dance champion, operates FollowMaxFomin studio in Montréal. He once came down in the top 24 competitors at the annual Blackpool Dance Festival in England.

**Brenton Mitchell** owns the Edgett Dance and Wellness studio in Halifax, Nova Scotia. He is the former Ten Dance Champion in Canada (2016-2017) and a Ten Dance finalist in the World Championship (2016) in Austria. He teaches along with **Jane Edgett**, a National Champion adjudicator and a Fellow of the U.K.-based Imperial Society of Teachers of Dancing (ISTD)and the CDF, and a six-instructor team.

**Michel Dubé**, owner of Michel & Company's studio in Halifax, is a former five-time champion of the Atlantic Ballroom dance competitions. Dubé has also finished at the top six twice at national competitions.

**Judy Knee**, a 45-year dance instructor, owns and operates The Judy Knee Dance Studio in St. John's, Newfoundland. Knee is a Fellow of both the ISTD and CDTA. In the 1970s, she was a winner of a scholarship awarded by the ISTD Ballroom Faculty. She specializes in the ballroom and the Latin dances as well as salsa and Argentine tango.

## Diverse Teachers in Social Ballroom/Latin

Not only are social dance teachers qualified by virtue of experience and or certification, but they also reflect the multicultural makeup of the communities they live in.

**Andy Wong**, a semi-retired Asian-Canadian dance instructor in Vancouver, operates The Grand Ballroom. It is now largely an online outlet for his video instruction material featuring him and two partners, one being his wife, Wendy. Wong and his wife had an unprecedented thirteen-year reign as British Columbia's amateur champions in both standard and Latin divisions and were finalists at the 1993 Canadian Championships.

**Zillion Wong, Faye Hung, Sarah Liang, Tony Fung, Mark Ma, Linda Zhang, Peter Chen, Laurie Xie** and **Angela Chu** are nine Asian-Canadians of the 12-instructor team at the Crystal Ballroom Studio, also in Vancouver.

**Steve Nelson** in Toronto is the first Black person to become a certified ballroom dance instructor in Canada and the first person of colour to be become a recognized dance adjudicator with the CDF. An independent, itinerant instructor, Nelson has taught at dozens of studios and social dance clubs over the past 30 years. He is a full member of the CDF, CDTA and the Canadian Dance and Dance Sport Council. He also became a Canadian roller champion—at age 13.

**Carlo** and **Monica Tran**, an Asian-Canadian couple, are principal instructors at the CM Cha Cha Cha Dance Studio in Markham, Ontario. Markham is home to 325,000 residents of whom more than 55 per cent are visible minorities. The Trans offer instruction in English, Cantonese and Mandarin.

**Robert Tang** and **Beverley Cayton-Tang** own DanceScape dance studio in Burlington, just southwest of Markham. Robert Tang is Asian-Canadian and Beverley was born in the U.K. Both were three-time Canadian and two-time North American Amateur Ballroom champions.

**Richard J. Thibault** is a fluently bilingual (French and English), independent instructor in Toronto. He hails from Rimouski, Québec. A licentiate of the Imperial Society of Teachers of Dancing in England, Thibault specializes in international Latin and standard as well as American rhythm and smooth dances. He is an adjudicator for the World Dance Organization and a fellow of Canada DanceSport.

**Arunas Bizokas** owns and operates Olympic Stars Dance Academy in Vaughan, Ontario. A Lithuanian-born ballroom dancer, he, with his partner, Katusha Demidova, won the World Championships title in 2009. In 2020 they were the reigning International, U.K. and British Professional Ballroom champions.

# The Salsa Dance Academy

Although the salsa education community in Canada has yet to develop a nationally recognized body to set standards and to promote exchange of knowledge, salsa instructors have learned from the world's best teachers through congresses here and in Latin American countries and in the U.S.

For instance, the 18th annual Canada Salsa & Bachata Congress—scheduled to be held in October of 2021 in Toronto—is chock-full of the world's most experienced teachers in the field. According to the organizers, 50 international artists, 70 dance companies from abroad and 45 "best instructors in the world" will be attending.

Other Canadian congresses—Montreal Salsa Convention, Calgary International Salsa Congress and the Vancity International Salsa Bachata Kizomba Festival (in British Columba)—have similar formats.

Let's look at the background of some Canadian salsa experts:

**Corey Solomon** and his team of **Samia Massoud** and **Jessica Sage**, operate the Dance 4U studio in Vancouver. Solomon and Jessica were born and raised in Canada and learned their craft locally and Sage is U.S.-born. They are known for their dedication to their game and doing the things in life they really love, such as salsa. Vancouver is commonly viewed as a salsa town where "students could go dancing six nights a week at various locations with a lot of nights having up to three locations running on the same night." Dance 4U's success has been to create "something unique and guaranteed fun" for their students.

**Ana Karen Lopez** and **Leonardo Lopez** (both formerly from Mexico) are salsa instructors at the Salsa Dance Explosion dance studio in Winnipeg. Ana Karen won the Pro-Am Canadian championships in Toronto and placed first at the Pro-Am World Salsa Championships in Miami. She is the founder of the first salsa for kids program in Winnipeg. Leonardo won a competition in Puerto Rican-style salsa in 1999 and has been teaching for sixteen years.

**Regan Hirose** and **Harold Rancon**, also in Winnipeg, have been World Bachata Cabaret champions nine times. They run the Dance World studio (formerly RHR Latin Dance Company), and have been teaching Salsa on 1, Salsa on 2 and Cuban salsa for a decade.

**Aleksander Saiyan** runs the Toronto Dance Salsa dance studio in north Toronto. He uses a three-prong strategy: "Entertain, educate and evolve." As a former unconfident, overweight young man who avoided attending dance clubs with friends, and suffering from hyperhydrosis (excessively sweaty palms), Aleks has evolved from being a feeble salsa student. He started in beginner classes and moved up to become an instructor and later appointed director of operations at Toronto Dance Salsa.

**Jennifer Aucoin** is co-owner of Steps Dance Studio in Toronto and co-founder of the Women's Salsa Retreat. A trained salsa judge, she has also adjudicated at a World Salsa Summit. She founded the annual four-day Canada Salsa & Bachata Congress. Her colleague, Angelo De Torres (studio co-owner), has trained with the world's best salsa teachers including Tito Ortos from whom he received his salsa certification. De Torres is a professional competitor and has won several competitions in the professional bachata division.

**Vanessa Stay**, who was born in Argentina, has owned Mississauga's Latin Energy Dance Company since 2002. She won the title of World Vice Champion at the Pro Classic Salsa championships in Miami and has been a judge for the World Latin Dance Cup event.

**Sandra Campanelli** runs Latin Groove Dance & Fitness on Montréal's Sainte-Catherine Street. It offers a trinity of dance services: it is a popular salsa dance studio combined with a 31-year-old Latin music band (*Sandra & the Latin Groove*) and also a booking agency for Latin artists. Campanelli is quadrilingual (French, English, Italian and Spanish). She receives rave reviews for her salsa teaching style.

**Adriano Ieropoli** and **Samantha Scali**, also in Montréal, founded Novaera Productions. The placed first in the 2017 World Salsa Summit in Miami.

**Trena Graham** owns Trenas Studio in Halifax. Well known for offering salsa workshops at Nova Scotia bachata dance festivals, Graham is also popular for her motto: "Stay focused on your dance goals but try not be stubborn about how you would achieve them," she maintains. "I don't know any [great dancers] who got to where they are exactly how they thought they could."


Despite the fact that many salsa dance venues are concentrated in Canada's biggest cities, many salsa instructors cannot make dance their full-time job—as enticing as that prospect would be. Many of them must still work in other occupations for their day jobs. Their night gigs are important fun for them as they try to meet the popular demand for social dancing instruction.

In Toronto, Canada's largest city, these highly skilled salsa teachers who have taught tens of thousands of *salseros* and s*alseras* over the years include Frank Bishun, Rene Delgado, Stephanie Gurnon, Jim Gronau, Abby Mina,

Oscar Naranjo, and Giovanni Torres.

In the past, these instructors taught at Greater Toronto venues such as Acrobat Lounge, Alleycatz, Ba-ba-lu-u's, Berlin Night Club, Copacabana, El Rancho (formerly El Borinquen), El Convento Rico, Fregata, La Bamba, La Classique, Latin Fever, Park Avenue, Plaza Flamingo, Six Degrees, Sparkles, and St. Paul's United Church.

(At the back of this book, you'll find listings of instructors and venues where salsa is taught.)

## Diverse Teachers in Salsa

Like the social ballroom faculty, those who teach salsa in Canada reflect a range of backgrounds—ethnic, social class and gender. Salsa teachers who were born outside Canada and immigrated here from the Caribbean and Latin America explain that the dance (and the music) have been part of their cultural heritage.

Others took up salsa after visiting Latin American countries and on returning home, learned the craft over time. They acquired their skills through group and private classes with the best instructors they could afford, as well as entering dance competitions.

(The professional salsa dance community has yet to organize and develop a nationally recognized body to exchange knowledge and to set standards of practice.)

A good example is Tania Wong, owner of and instructor at Tania Dance Connexion in the extremely multicultural city of Toronto. Wong, an Asian-Canadian, has won various world and national competitions. She is a three-time Canadian Bachata Champion, was second runner up at the World Bachata Championship and has been "Toronto Salsa Champion" multiple times.

Many social ballroom instructors also teach salsa to their ballroom students who wish to visit salsa clubs for new dance experiences. For example, Vancouver's Dance 4U's owner Corey Solomon and his instructors U.S.-born Sarnia Massoud and Canadian-born Jessica Sage teach social ballroom but due to a big demand for salsa has almost exclusively turned to salsa teaching. Solomon said: "for business, when every eight out of ten phone calls … are [students] looking for some salsa dance lessons—it only made sense to make the change."

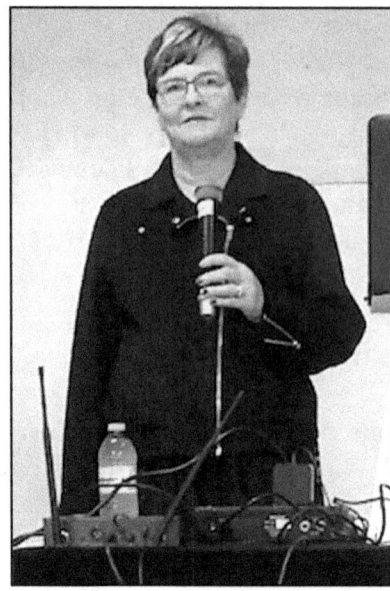

Figure 9: Saskatchewan square dancing caller Linda Gilchrist with her microphone at a Swan Valley Hoedowners party.

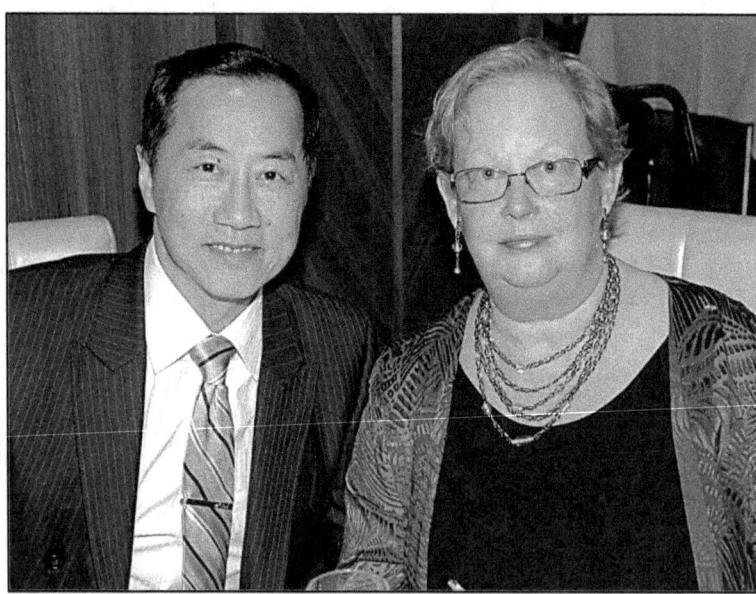

Figure 10: Semi-retired B.C. instructors Andy and Wendy Wong at their Grand Ballroom studio in Vancouver.

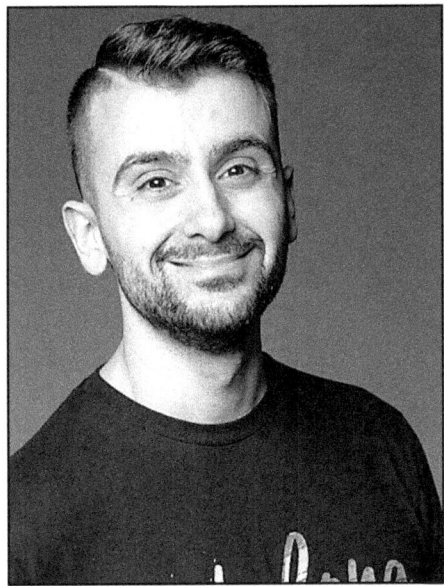

Figure 11: Educate, entertain and evolve," says Toronto Dance Salsa studio's Aleks Saiyan.

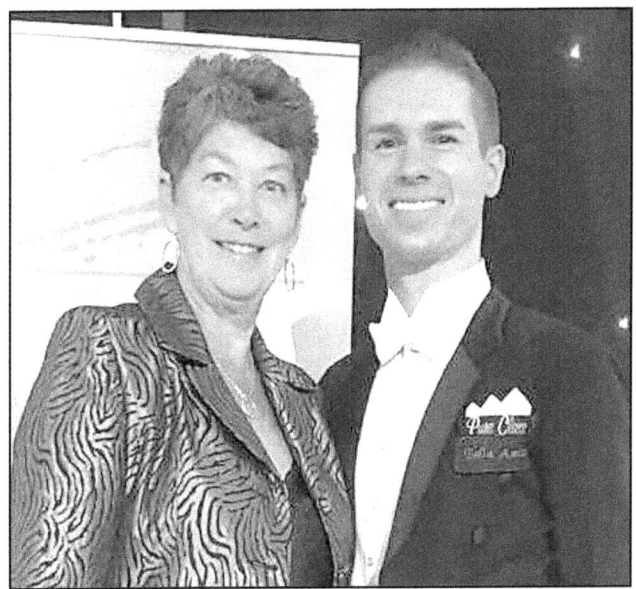

Figure 12: Nova Scotian instructors Brenton Mitchell and Jane Edgett at the Edgett Dance & Wellness Dance School in downtown Halifax.

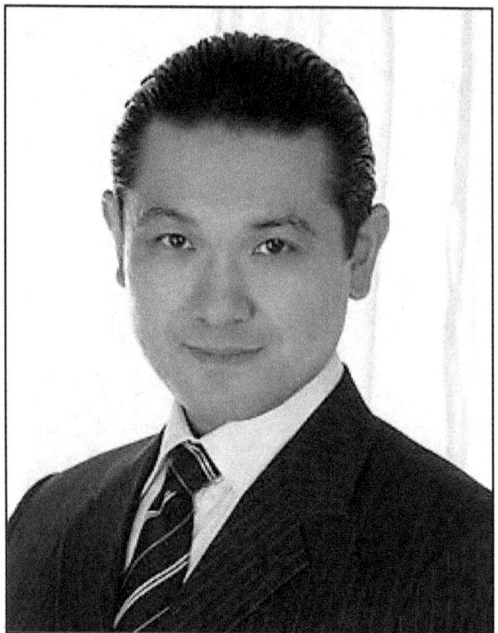

Figure 13: Long-time Argentine tango instructor Leo Sato in Calgary.

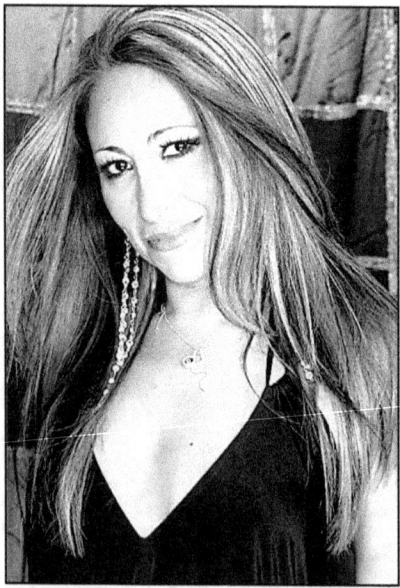

Figure 14: In Montreal, Sandra Campanelli, owner of Latin Groove Dance Studio gets rave reviews for salsa teaching.

# The Argentine Tango Dance Academy

Unlike the social ballroom and salsa dance scene, the Argentine tango community has a relatively low profile. Tens of thousands of participants, however, pursue this dance.

For many social dancers of all disciplines, it had been difficult to know where *milongas* (tango parties and dances) were in any town. They were usually few and far in between. However, with the World Wide Web, social dancers have a much easier time accessing information.

The tango's profile is growing wider each year with tango festivals. In these settings, tango dancers become more familiar with and learn from the *crème de la crème* in this dance art.

Unlike the salsa congresses and ballroom dancesport competitions, Argentine tango festivals (such as Toronto Tango Festival or the Toronto Tango 8 Festival) may mask the depth of talent among the Canadian community. The few tango festivals generally feature foreign-based experts so the local pool of teachers can update their knowledge and skills.

Nonetheless, home-grown Canadian talent in Argentine tango is abundant:

**Gabriel Monty** has been teaching tango for more than 30 years and operates Vancouver's Argentine Tango Lab. He has competed in the World Tango Championship in salon tango (*tango de Pista*) and stage tango (*tango escenario*),.and performed in well known milongas in Buenos Aires.

**Patricia** and **Bobbi Lusic** are co-directors and instructors who run the TangoBug studio in the Greater Vancouver area. Bobbi Lusic is examination secretary for the ballroom and specialty dances division of the British Columbia chapter of the Canadian Dance Teachers' Association, and she is a licentiate in the same dance division. They base their teaching on a "four stages of mastery" approach" In their words, these are "distinct stages through which all human beings progress whenever they learn anything new."

**Leo Sato** is a tango instructor in Calgary for twenty years and has produced three Live Tango Shows for Calgary residents. He has performed with dance partner Marina Gonzales and Angela Mulrooney of Unleashed Dance Company, and the Calgary Philharmonic Orchestra on themed evenings. He was a finalist in Colombia's 2017 Open Salon Tango Championship Senior division. In the world of cinematography, he choreographed two movies: *The Lost Tango 2003* and the British blockbuster *Burn-Up* (2007).

**Elizabeth Sadowska** is not only a tango *maestra* in her own right as owner of Rhythm & Motion Dance Studio in Toronto, but she is also an accomplished ballroom dance competitor. Sadowska has organized annual Tango Marathons. She teaches all styles of Argentine tango including close embrace, open, salon, *milonguero* and *nuevo*. She and her instructors are still remembered for performing at the opening ceremonies of the 2015 Pan-American games and staging the first Tango Short Film & Documentary Festival in North America.

**Andrea Shepherd** and **Wolfgang Mercado-Alatrista** are the owners, teachers and artistic directors at MonTango in Montréal since 2018. They have been dancing together eighteen years. Their approach to the art blends both traditional and modern tango techniques and they displayed this mix at the 2013 Festival International de Tango de Montréal. Both also won first place in a three-dance event in the professional category, at the Chic de la Danse competition.

**Lorne Buick** and **Martina Sommer** teach at the You, Two, Can Tango! dance studio in Halifax. This studio is a happy hunting ground for Nova Scotians who are into Argentine tango dancing. Both Buick and Sommer are also certified senior fitness instructors. Not only have they trained hundreds of students, but they have also successfully introduced tango as a tool for rehabilitation and health promotion in vulnerable populations, such as those with Parkinson's disease. Their regular "Tea & Tango" program, incorporating dance for persons with Parkinson's, has been viewed as "a first in Canada."

## Diverse Teachers in Argentine Tango

To meet the demand for Argentine tango lessons, Canadian Argentine dance studios have scouted for the best tango teachers in the world. Instructors have traveled far and wide to places like Argentina, the United Kingdom and Asia to further their training.

Foreign instructors are often invited to lead workshops. Plus, Canadian-born instructors lend their expertise around the world as well. All of this is so the instructors of the dance academies can become more effective teachers.

Four experienced instructors are good examples of this international training and experience.

**Lina Chan**, a former Hong Kong dancer and teacher, is an experienced *tanguera* and teacher of more than thirty-five years. She joined forces with **Bulent Karabagli** at the Bulent + Lina tango studio in Toronto.

**Karabagli** himself has thirty years of experience teaching and dancing tango around the world as guest "master" in major festivals and cities in Canada, the United States and as far as Europe. The studio usually runs the Tango8Fest and Marathon.

**Egor Belashov**, formerly of northwestern Russia, is a 2008 Canadian professional (American style) ballroom champion who trained in tango to meet his students' demand for Argentine tango. His Dance With Me studios located in Toronto and Markham (Ontario) provide group and private classes.

**Estelle Nicol** is a highly trained instructor and has been teaching since 2006. She is Toronto-born and a co-founder of City Dance Corps in Toronto. She developed an innovative hybrid dance that fuses salsa with tango. Experts in the field recognize her experience and innovative style and have invited her to run master workshops and choreography in Bermuda, Israel, Italy and Greece.

# The Volunteer-based Square Dance and Round Dance Academy

Where there is square dancing in Canada, there might also be round dancing. As well, there could be contra dancing, line dancing or clogging included (which are beyond the scope of this book).

(Contra dancing or *contredanse* evolved from English country dances that were imported into Canada centuries ago; please see Chapter One of this book. Clogging is a dance using clogging footwear to strike the heel, the toe, or both against the dance floor. Line dancing is a dance for individuals who repeat the choreographed steps of various dance forms with all dancers.)

Square dance is a country dance involving four couples in a square or sometimes a circle, depending on one's geographic location. The dancers are prompted by a caller who acts like a master of ceremonies and selects the dance steps and may instruct when necessary.

Round dancing is choreographed ballroom dances for couples, who follow the instructions of a "cuer'" to progress in a circular, counter-clockwise pattern around a dance floor. Many square dance clubs have "round dancing" as part of their legal name and therefore mandate round dancing activities as a key program for members.

The Canadian Square & Round Dance Society is the national umbrella organization coordinating the services of the provincial square and round dance federations. The federations, in turn, are the frontline hubs that serve a network of clubs in various geographic "zones" in the provinces. (In Nova Scotia, zones are referred to as "cultural regions.")

Because callers, leaders, cuers and, to some extent, musicians such as fiddlers and deejays, collectively form the backbone of the talent pool that support dancers, some zones have set up "associations", or coordinating groups, of callers, instructors and even dancers.

The cadre of square dance providers is professional in the sense that they have professional level skills but are largely acting as volunteers in Canada.

According to Jerry Jestin, a professional square dance caller and round dance cuer in Red Deer County, Alberta, who retired his microphone in December 2019, "[t]here are very few people worldwide that make their living from this," he says in an email. "I flew over 3.5 million miles travelling to engagements since late '70s."

Bud Sedman and Brenda Ryder, co-presidents of the Alberta Square & Round Dance Federation, concur. Sedman says that he is aware of only two people in Canada who do this and get paid.

The Manitoba federation describes these experts as "… the wonderful leaders that call, cue and instruct for the Federation Clubs." It announces on its website that "without them there would be no dancing."[4]

For instance, within the seven zones of the Alberta Square & Round Dance Federation zones, there are five associations of callers. Furthermore, the provincial federation also contains two associations for dancers, one for cuers and one for instructors.

Here's a look at the approximate number of callers and cuers across the country in 2020:

- British Columbia listed 61 callers and cuers.
- In Alberta, there were 44 callers, cuers and leaders. Instructors in that province are represented by the Square and Round Dance Instructors Association of Alberta, which is headed by Dave Littlefair.
- Saskatchewan had 26 callers, cuers and instructors.
- Manitoba had 15 callers and cuers.
- Ontario had 79 callers and cuers.
- Québec had 144 callers and cuers.
- New Brunswick had 20 callers and cuers. The New Brunswick federation has paired with Prince Edward Island to form the NB and PEI Callers' Association with Roger and Anna Sherren as its "president couple."

- Nova Scotia had 34 leaders among its eight cultural regions. These leaders are members of the Association of Nova Scotia Square and Round Dance Teachers. The association, in turn, supports the activities of the Maritime Callers and Cuers Association.
- Prince Edward Island had two callers.
- Newfoundland-Labrador – the federation was inactive in 2020.

## Olde Tyme Square Dancing and Modern Square Dancing

As the heavy snows began to slowly melt during the winter of 1954, the first executive board of the Toronto-based Canadian Olde Tyme Square Dance Association decided to have its first spring dance.

According to its then president, James Fisher, the goal was "to promote the traditional dances, with ties and roots reaching back to our forefathers, along with the best of the new ones."

Explaining the difference between the traditional square dance and the modern Western square dancing espoused by the Canadian Square and Round Dance Society, Judy Greenhill, a modern square dance instructor in Ontario, says the modern version "is organized differently, whereas 'olde tyme' square dancing is open dancing."

In olde tyme dancing, "anyone can go at any time and they can sort of pick it up by watching or listening, or maybe going to an introductory class," says Greenhill.

In modern square dance, however, "you'd have to take lessons and it's divided into lessons and there are nine levels altogether," she says.

Modern square dancers require a "huge commitment." Because the instruction is "so codified … the only way to get anything new is to master a level and go on and learn the next level".

By contrast, Greenhill, the instructor for Royal City Squares in Guelph, Ontario, says old-time square dancers tend "to want more instant gratification."

Olde tyme dance caller Ralph Price and his wife, , of Horseshoe Valley in Ontario, has this rejoinder: "Modern square dancing … doesn't have the same spark …. [W]ith the modern, you don't necessarily have to listen [to the caller who prompts the dance] because it's all choreographed as to what you're doing."

"In olde tyme, you've got to listen to me [as the caller], and I'm not [calling] the same thing every time," Price explains.

Ontario olde tyme square dancer Hindy Bornstein says the modern dancers are so focused on what they learn in classes. In the modern genre, "it seems like you don't have a lot of evenings or afternoons where it's just a dance."

Bornstein continues: "You go to your [modern square dance] club every week and you learn the movements, but in olde tyme, it's the opposite—you could walk in off the street, come to a dance and we would get up and dance because you know your right hand from your left hand."

Bornstein says it is not that she is against "learning." She emphasizes that learning is just more front and centre in the modern square dance experience: "In modern, you can't begin to imagine what the movements mean from hearing words. So, you have to learn them. They're different depending on where you're standing.

"If you're standing at the top of the square or at the side of the square or at the bottom, the movements will be different at the same call."

Toronto's Bill Russell, 2021 president of the Canadian Olde Tyme Square Dance Association, says it's easier dancing olde tyme because "generally, callers will explain the figures - where you go - depending on the experience of the dancers. Most dancers do not do any special steps while dancing.".

## Facing the Future—Two National Square Dance Associations

Both national associations of modern Western square dance and "olde tyme" are currently suffering from lower membership levels, compared to previous years. And it is not primarily due to the 2020-2021 pandemic.

Eric McCormack, a former six-year president of the Canadian Square and Round Dance Society, notes that the state of the dance is not very good. "Oh, it's actually shrinking," he admits. "Mostly it's because [most members] have just gotten too old to dance or they can't travel at night."

The age factor also affects membership in the olde tyme square dancing association. Dance caller Ralph Price agrees, admitting that "most participants are 65 or older."

"Our main concern is that we can't get the young people involved. They look at it as an old people's recreation," says McCormack who is still active at the national level.

He says some provincial federations have embarked on initiatives to reverse the declining membership trend. He points out that "in B.C. they do get involved with competitive dancing across the border [like] between Washington State and B.C. and, and when there's no pandemic, that seems to be working really well, trying to figure out ways to get the kids involved.

"We're working a lot with the Americans because their organizations are having the same problem," says McCormack. "So, we're working a lot with them to try and develop something, to get people involved."

McCormack also points out that modern square dance groups, notably in New Brunswick and Québec, hold afternoon dance events to try and improve membership levels.

In the meantime, the olde tyme association is trying to survive, especially with the protracted pandemic. "We're really stalled," says its Toronto-based president Bill Russell. "We have a limited amount of resources that have been passed on to be used, like old amplifiers, books and recordings … we have members who don't really use computers," Russell says.

One of the bright spots is that the olde tyme association has been encouraging its callers and dancers to organize activities that would keep the olde tyme brand alive. Russell points to examples such as participation in the annual Royal Agricultural Winter Fair olde tyme dance competition, and the events usually held in Dundalk and Pancake Hill in Ontario.

(In February 2021, the board of directors of the Winter Fair announced that it plans to open in the autumn. The fair was cancelled in 2020 due to the pandemic.)

Ralph Price is one of these bright spot organizers. During the 2020-2021 pandemic, he organized dance events right on his home driveway in Horseshoe Valley, Ontario.

# Municipal 'Leisure Services'—A Social Dance Academy

For more than fifty years, British Columbia's North Vancouver Recreation & Culture Commission, has actively encouraged "active healthy lifestyles and recreational pursuits for its 52,000 residents.

Similarly, Newmarket located north of Toronto, also actively organizes and implements recreational activities for its 89,000 residents through initiatives such as its long-term 2015-2025 *Recreation Playbook*—described as a master plan to support a broader more ambitious *Cultural Master Plan*.

In doing so, both municipalities have—and continue—to run social dance classes in salsa, Argentine tango and social ballroom for the young and old. These are among the dozens of leisure activities they sponsor, with their leisure services (often called 'parks and rec') department taking the lead.

(During the 2020-2021 pandemic, the two local governments as well as dozens of Canadian municipalities canceled in-person dance classes.)

To run these programs, the departments hire part-time instructors as employees or as independent contractors. These instructors can be competitive dancers, independent private instructors, or teachers from dance studios.

This strategy reduced the cost of having full-time professionals on the payroll. Plus, taxpayer-funded infrastructure such as high-quality buildings with well-maintained amenities such as heat and air conditioning, already exist. Municipal services therefore ensure residents can physically and financially access dance services more easily.

# Author's 2018-2019 Survey of Social Dance Classes

The author emailed a three-question survey to 112 urban, suburban and rural municipalities in Canada about social dance classes in their recreation department between 2018 and 2019 and the participation rates of residents.

## Overall Response

Fifty-two municipalities responded to the survey (46%). Of the 52 respondents, 21 or close to three-quarters (40%) offered dance classes during the period surveyed. The rest (60%) reported they did not offer social dance classes during 2018-2019.

## The Questions

1) What are the registration numbers for 2018 and 2019?
2) Please comment on the demographics of participants?
3) Please reflect on your city's experience in providing the service?

## Details of Responses

The names and registration numbers of the 21 responding municipalities that offered social dance classes were:

| Year | Registration Year | Registration #s |
|---|---|---|
| **Over 100,000 residents** | | |
| Belleville | 2018 | 86 |
| | 2019 | 110 |
| Cambridge | 2018 | 124 |
| | 2019 | 100 |
| Edmonton | 2018 | 5 classes |
| | 2019 | 4 classes*** |
| Halifax | 2018 | 65 |
| | 2019 | 268+ |
| Kitchener | 2018 | 16 |
| | 2019 | 16** |
| Toronto | 2018 | 324 |
| | 2019 | 257 |
| Windsor | 2018 | 43 |
| | 2019 | 105^^^ |
| **50,000 to 99,999 residents** | | |
| Caledon | 2018 | 048 |
| | 2019 | 16 |
| Maple Ridge | 2018 | 148 |
| | 2019 | 127 |
| Newmarket | 2018 | 105 |
| | 2019 | 70 |
| North Vancouver | 2018 | 324 |
| | 2019 | 257 |
| **Under 50,000 residents** | | |
| Bradford/West Gwillimbury | 2018 | 103 |
| | 2019 | 59<<<< |
| East Gwillimbury | 2018 | 1500* |
| | 2019 | 1600* |
| Joliette | 2018 | 240 |
| | 2019 | 240++ |
| King | 2018 | 12 |
| | 2019 | 31 |
| Lake Country | 2018 | 9 classes |
| | 2019 +++ | 2 classes |
| Pointe-Claire | 2018 | 69 |
| | 2019 | 69 < |

| Year | Registration Year | Registration #s |
|---|---|---|
| Salmon Arm | 2018 | 123 |
| | 2019 | 123^ |
| Val-des-Monts | 2018 | 0 |
| | 2019 | 41<< |
| Westmount | 2018 | 162 |
| | 2019 | 162^^ |
| Whitchurch-Stouffville | 2018 | 24 |
| | 2019 | 24<<< |

**Legend**
- \* Mainly children's social dance programs.
- \*\* Mainly seniors in age group 60s to 70s.
- \*\*\* Fill rate of 89 and 78% respectively.
- + Only includes adults in social dance, line dance, jive fox trot and belly dance.
- ++ Registrants are 60-80 years old.
- +++ For levels 1 and 2.
- ^ Numbers are distributed through 8 classes and 4 open houses during 2018-2019.
- ^^ Numbers relate to one session. Three classes offered only on Mondays and Thursdays.
- ^^^ 2018 featured only one Fall session.
- < 4 social dance classes and 3 Argentine tango classes.
- << No courses offered in 2018.
- <<< Ballroom classes were cancelled due to lack of registration; numbers reflect line dance.
- <<<< Fall of 2019 figure not provided.

## Commentary on the Demographics of Participants During 2018-2019

- **City of Belleville:** "The ages are all over—from early 20s to late 70s. The average ages are between 55-65."
- **Town of Bradford West Gwillimbury:** 72 per cent of 103 dance registrations in 2018 were over 50 years of age; 73 percent of 105 registrations in 2019 were over 50 years.

- **Town of Caledon:** "We don't have [information] on the demographics of participants."
- **Town of East Gwillimbury:** "The Town does not track demographics of participants...."
- **City of Edmonton:** "We don't have records of demographic information ... our classes do have a separate bar code for registration so [we] can balance partner leaders and followers."
- **City of Joliette:** "Participants are, on average, between 60 and 80 years old."
- **Township of King:** "The majority of the participants are between 60-75 years of age."
- **City of Kitchener:** "... [C]omprising ... couples ... in their sixties and seventies."
- **City of Maple Ridge**: "Demographics are mainly couples aged 45-65."
- **Town of Newmarket**: "Clients have been between 25 and 60 years of age from a broad range of cultures. The average female dancer is between 35 and 60. Good mix of couples, and quite a few singles.

"Many participants had been looking for extracurricular activities for themselves and their partners, to enjoy the exercise and social opportunity. Some clients were wanting to learn the basics and continue to enjoy socially. What the instructor had done was exceptional—he organized a trip following each course for folks having completed the course to enjoy dancing at a dance club in the city.

"Ballroom dance can enhance overall successful aging by promoting long-standing participation in physical and social activities. Ballroom dance is dancing movement patterns. These dances include the international-style standard dances such as the slow fox trot, the two waltzes, tango and the international-style Latin American dances like the rumba, samba and cha-cha-cha.

"Ballroom dance, as serious leisure, is a core leisure activity. It is so gratifying that its participants orchestrate a set of activities that progressively increase their knowledge, skills, and overall participation in the activity and shared experience."

- **City of Toronto**: In 2018, there were 28,288 registrations in dance programs—covering different dance forms—of which 24,339 were in arts-based programs and 3,949 were in fitness-based programs. (Dance programs fall under arts programs and fitness programs). Registrations for *arts-based* programs by demographic groups: early years (0-5) - 12,012; child (6-12) 3,289; child/youth (6-12) - 52; youth (13-24) - 540; adults (18-59) - 2,318; and older adults (60+) - 6,128. (*Fitness-based* demographics not included.)

In 2019, there were 28,340 registrations in dance programs of which 24,393 were in arts-based programs and 3,947 in fitness-based programs. Registrations for *arts-based* programs by demographic groups: early years (0-5) - 11,970; child (6-12)- 3.445; child/youth - 52; youth (13-24) - 379; adults (18-59) - 2,269; and older adults (60+) - 6,278. (*Fitness-based* demographics not included.)

- **City of Windsor:** In 2018, "most participants were in their 30s, with another group in their 60s, there were a few 18-year-olds. In 2019, the average age of participants here was 43, with many participants in their 50s and 60s."
- **Town of Whitchurch-Stouffville**: "Participants in the social classes tend to be female aged 65-75."
- **Municipality of Val-des-Monts**: 17 men and 24 women registered; the majority were in the age range of 50s to 60s.

## Experience in Providing Dance Services

- **City of Belleville:** "Some seasons are more popular than others. We offer a beginner class and an intermediate class each week. There has been no demand for increasing that number of classes offered. We accept 24 people in each class."
- **Town of Bradford West Gwillimbury:** "Provided an opportunity for adult participation. Dancing has been offered for a number of years."
- **Town of East Gwillimbury**: "As the Town's population is aging and looking for ways to be active and healthy, we have seen an increase in requests from adults and older adults for ballroom dancing. Our children's recreational dance classes population has increased as well for recreational purposes."
- **City of Edmonton:** "We know our classes are an opportunity for people to connect with fellow Edmontonians at a community hub (our recreation centres). This allows us to bring our programming to different quadrants of the City of Edmonton, making our offering more

accessible for patrons. Dance is also an opportunity to focus on overall health as it's an active mode of recreation."

- **Township of King**: "We were very happy to see the increase of participants from 2018-2019. The participants really enjoyed the instructor and the progression of the class. The program is open for all skill levels and does not require for [anyone] to have a partner. This was a fun way for our seniors to interact with each other and have a fun social class."
- **City of Kitchener:** "This service has been very well received and appreciated by the various couples that attend. Its social connections are most rewarding, not to mention the benefits of physical dancing."
- **City of Joliette:** "We have been doing this activity for several years since we know how much it is appreciated by participants. More than 80 seniors get together every week to participate in this activity."
- **City of Maple Ridge**: "The classes are well received. We have been running them for almost 20 years. We also offer Friday Night Dance classes (twice a month) for students to continue practice or for the community to come and try dance. They receive a one-hour lesson and an additional two hours of practice time. The bar is open to allow for a more social evening. On average we have 35-40 students come out on Fridays for some fun."
- **Town of Newmarket:** "Over the past ten years this program has been offered on an ongoing basis, ever since I [Janis Luttrell] have had care of arts and culture programs for the municipality. The program is one I consider to be essential to the roster of programs provided to the adult participants.

  "The ballroom Latin dance program delivered by our instructor, John Yuen, has received stellar reviews from regular follow up, as expressed by customers directly. We receive consistently positive feedback about how well enjoyed it is. He is an especially great teacher which makes the program the success it has been. Since we began, we have built three levels of programming delivery which allows for a continuous learning experience which our customers love."
- **City of Pointe-Claire**: "The City . . . stands out for its very diversified range of services, in all spheres of activity (aquatic, nautical, physical, cultural). Social dance classes are part of [the] desire to continually

reach a larger audience. The lessons are appreciated and the teachers are very qualified."

- **City of Salmon Arm:** "Our organization has on occasion hosted a Registered Program for teaching dance to local residents, but the numbers are likely less than 100 over the past 5 years."
- **City of Toronto**: "Dance programs fall under two main categories in our Community Recreation offerings: Arts programs and Fitness programs.
    - "…[D]ance programs provide opportunities for participants to learn and develop new skills and techniques, as well as participate in physical and social activity across all age groups, especially with our senior population.
    - "The programs allow participants to experience different genres of dance at an introductory level with the opportunity to move forward and pursue higher skill development in a respective genre.
    - "City of Toronto dance programs provide City staff with an opportunity to contribute their skills, talents, knowledge and expertise to engaging and teaching residents as well as helping Toronto communities flourish."
- **City of Windsor:** "Participants and the instructor were extremely passionate about dancing. Overall, the reception for these programs has been very positive and many adults enjoy the opportunity to learn the new dance skills while also experiencing the class with a friend or significant other."
- **Municipality of Val-des-Monts**: <Nous notons une croissance dans le nombre de participants. L'activité est appréciée. Nous avons un bon service de la contratuelle offrant le cours pour la Municipalité. Malheuresement, la croissance d'activité dans notre programmation est directement liée aux locaux disponibles. Ainsi, malgré la bonne participation, nous ne pouvons pas développer advantage de cours similaires sans venir au détriment de d'autres.>
    - *Translation:* "We are observing a growth in the number of participants. This is appreciated. We have a good contract service offering the course for the municipality. Unfortunately, the growth of activity in our programming depends on facilities being available.

So, despite the good participation, we cannot develop additional related courses at the expense of others."
- **Town of Whitchurch-Stouffville**: "We have had little interest in couple dance classes; on a social basis, however, dance-themed individual classes to increase physical activity are quite popular."

# Indie Instructors at Volunteer-run Dance Clubs

As a child, Juliana Chow began dancing with ballet. Today, as an adult, she does social ballroom dancing—international-style tango being her favourite--at the University of British Columbia Dance Club (UBCDC). Established in 1949, it is one of the oldest university ballroom dance clubs in Canada.

Elected in 2020 for a one-year term as president of the club, she and her fourteen volunteer executives often registered for dance classes that were held in the Great Hall of the university's Nest Building every semester. Dance registration fees cover instructors' expenses.

The club's four dance instructors come from outside the university and belong to an elite group of B.C. ballroom dance champions; some are former members of the club they now teach at. Two instructors, a husband-and-wife team, Clara Shih-Marasigan and Joel Marasigan, for instance, were dance partners in the club during the 1990s and today run a successful private studio—JC Dance Co. in Vancouver.

Likewise, the 30-Up Club, an incorporated social club in Toronto's west end, hosts a variety of occasional instructors. Its staple services are the weekend night dances that attract hundreds of ballroom dancers from the city as well as from afar.

Like the UBCDC, the instructors are not club employees but independent contractors running exclusive events for group lessons or teaching at small dance parties, such as the Sunday afternoon "tea dances" and special "themed" nights. Instructors from the Greater Toronto Area, such as Mary Adams, Sylvain Cardinal, Mandy Epprecht, Konstantine Antonov, Patricia Goh, Deniz Karakulak, Stilian Kostov, Derek Krzyszkowksi, Larry Hall, Phil Lee, Steve Murgatroyd, Steve Nelson, Richard J. Thibault, and Marla Vetesse, have passed through the club doors.

Many of them still teach there. Steve Nelson holds a "Wednesday night dance". Konstantine Antonov is a regular; he has even been running a virtual event during the COVID-19 pandemic.

Reflecting on the many separate independent activities within the 30-Up

Club, Marjorie White, the president, suggests "the 30-Up hosts clubs within our club."

## 'Helping Out' the Social Clubs

The first migrations of indie instructors from private studios to university and community social clubs were inevitable. Once clubs decided to open, they had to rely on outside help "to spread the joy of dancing," according to Fred Cheng, University of Waterloo Ballroom & Latin Club president.

Furthermore, university and social dance clubs need to hire outside instructors because their board of directors are dance enthusiasts, not dance professionals.

In Cheng's club, the need for importing outside instructors became urgent four years ago when his executive team decided to enter dancesport competitions in the United States. Cheng, along with his vice-president of finance Kyra McEllistrum, and other executive members spend time helping dancers, but outside expert instructors such as Mandy Epprecht were a godsend for proper training in competitive work.

Another reason private sector instructors teach at social clubs is because they have spaces in their schedules that allow them to teach outside the studios they own or rent. As well, they increase their reach in the market and, of course, revenue.

The UW Swing Club at the University of Waterloo provides opportunities to learn American social dances from the 1900s (lindy hop, Charleston, Balboa, shag). It, too, relies on six outside instructors to carry out its mandate which is "to help students get exposed to swing dancing and related styles of dance, encourage an active and social lifestyle and ultimately, connect the dance community on campus to the ones in the larger Kitchener-Waterloo area."

For Canada's dozens of university, commercial and volunteer-run social dance clubs, access to imported instructor help has never been more important.

## Conclusion

The dance academies for the four social dance forms described in this book—as well as the dozens of others not covered in this book—represent the heart of Canada's robust social dance industry. Feeding into this industry is a supply chain of domestic and international companies such as shoe designers and manufacturers, cobblers, producers of dance educational materials (DVDs, music CDs and books), orchestras and swag promotional item makers.

The operators of Canadian social dance studios are generally small-business people. Most of them lease space to run their dance classes. Those who run the largest studios have unusually spacious ballroom dance spaces—7,000 square feet, for example. Some studios would usually divide large spaces into "studios" of various sizes and sublet for dance practice and events.

Although the Florida-based Arthur Murray International Inc. operates twenty franchised studios in Canada, Canadian dancers have dozens of other options to choose from, depending on where they live. The largest cities such as Montreal, Vancouver and Toronto usually have more than fifty studios. Appendix 2, at the back of the book, outlines the names of hundreds of dance studios and instructors from coast to coast as well as square and round dance clubs.

Dance schools and independent instructors compete for fee-paying customers. Like universities, grocery stores and financial advisors, only the better ones thrive while others may just hang by a thread.

For many social dance consumers, "better" means not just loyalty to an individual instructor and her expertise, but also the perception they have of the instructor's comportment: that is, the degree to which she shows genuine interest in helping dancers achieve their objectives. Other qualities that consumers look for include honesty, compassion for and respect shown to them.

In addition to registration and studio subletting fees—their primary source of revenue—studios boost sales by cross-selling dance-related products through their website and social media. Merchandise includes branded products (T-shirts, outerwear, coffee mugs, replacement soles for shoes) with the fastest moving items being dance shoes, music CDs, dance DVDs, books, and attire for men and women.

During the COVID-19 pandemic in 2020-2021, the financial losses incurred due to lockdowns caused a few dance studios to permanently close their doors. Even some volunteer-run square dancing clubs did so.

Some studio owners, while waiting for the third wave of the pandemic to recede, have turned to related pursuits, such as wellness and yoga training, to survive. And online classes continue unabated.

The author's municipal survey found that most social dance registrants in municipal "parks and rec" departments tend to be persons in their early years, children, adults and older adults. In the case of privately owned studios, younger people (16-40 age group) tend to be the major registrants, according to Mississauga, Ont.-based instructor Mandy Epprecht, who has been teaching for more than thirty years.

In the meantime, while the pandemic's current wave is at its height in most places, the leisure services planners in municipalities that offer social dance classes, are waiting with bated breath to reopen their dance.

# Appendix A: "The 39 Opinions" on competitive dancing, a representation of social dance

**Anonymous.** Caledon, Ontario. "It's clear how much skill, practice and preparation (physical and mental) are needed for any type of competition, including ballroom dancing competitions."

**Minoo Asgary,** Toronto. "I love it. I love the women's dance sequences. I wish I could do them. And that's going to be me."

**Larry Clark,** Halifax, Nova Scotia. "The first word that comes to my mind when I look at competitive dancing is 'regimental.' It's so precise, and it's almost regimental in appearance. I look at it and it's beautiful …. The beautiful costumes, but it's not really reality for me and Marg [my wife] because of our age. Because it's for show, it doesn't look like it's for enjoyment."

**Ruth Daccord** (educational assistant), Bradford West Gwillimbury. "I love watching competitive dancing. Hours of intense and consistent practice coupled with beautiful outfits, music and impeccable timing—all put together, it looks stunning."

**Maria Dobrynina,** Newmarket, Ontario. "I get a lot of pleasure seeing the process of professionals dancing—wearing beautiful costumes and moving to great music at the same time. It's like beholding art and experiencing many positive emotions at the same time."

**Sue Edney,** Calgary. "It's very elegant and graceful. I enjoy watching it. It brings back memories. We used to have a ballroom dancing neighbour with whom I once had a dance."

**Donna Flatman,** Salmon Arm, British Columbia. "It is a pleasure to watch high levels of dance and to learn a little about dance technique through the judges' feedback. Watching how the amateurs [on the *Dancing with the Stars* TV show] become accomplished dancers is inspirational."

**Brooklyn Foley,** Calgary. Alberta. "When I see those shows, I think about how I can't do it, and how I am uncoordinated. I definitely admire them, though. It's not my forte and I wish I could do what they do."

**Jim Forde,** Calgary Police Force (Retired), Calgary. "I am amazed how you can take a celebrity who normally doesn't dance ballroom-style and turn him or her, with practice into a competitive dancer. It just goes to show that with proper instruction and the will to learn to do something, you can do it very well. What I like about it is the grace and beauty of two people dancing to the music using a tremendous dance form."

**William Gibzey,** Bradford West Gwillimbury, Ontario. "I do not watch it because I believe it is an act and not dancing; their moves are professional and have been practised a million times just like acrobats. Their costumes do not impress me because they do not apparently pay for them, the studio [sponsoring a show like *Dancing with the Stars*] picks up all their tabs."

**Sandra Holliday-Tucker,** Newmarket. "It's magical to watch. ... years of practice appearing to be so effortless."

**Veronica Holly,** Tillsonburg, Ontario "When I see them dancing, I wish I could do that. It's beautiful to look at. The dancers make it look so easy to do. But you know if that's your profession, you should be able to do it well and make it look like it's easy to do, when it's not."

**Omar Kazi,** Toronto. "I love the choreography each couple comes up with."

**Nella Keating,** Newmarket. "I love watching them do the figures. What it does for me, as a dancer, is that it inspires to get my own dancing figures right. I do love the costumes. Some of the ladies' costumes are gorgeous. Watching professional dancers inspires me to continue dancing."

**Patrick Keating,** Newmarket. "The thing that strikes me or where I find it really interesting is the precision with which they do some of the movements—whether they be something very sharp and quick, or even if it's just a slow drawing in [of some body part] kind of thing. Also, you can just tell from the expression of their face of their dedication. It sort of inspires me a bit."

**Kelvin Lee,** Calgary. "I always thought it is one of those things that is very graceful. Coming from someone like me who isn't coordinated or graceful with my limbs, I think it's amazing that they can do what they do."

**Dale Lubberts,** East Gwillimbury, Ontario. "It's not realistic because it is a one-time performance. People who dance professionally go from competition to competition, they really know ballroom dancing!"

**Jelies J. Lubberts**, East Gwillimbury. "Competitive dancing is a good thing, provided it is friendly and fair."

**Flori Mackie**, Bradford West Gwillimbury, Ontario. "What I see doesn't appear to fun at all—not to me anyway. The dance moves are very regimented, very precise with no margin for flexibility or errors or improvising. The tension between the dance partners is palpable. To me this kind of dancing is just too serious, it lacks laughter and spontaneity."

**Pat Mastrandrea**, Newmarket. "It takes a lot of guts, a lot of training. I mean, you know, it takes a good part of their life. They need to contribute to achieve those results in competitive dancing. I have a friend who competes in world competitions and she's an awesome dancer. Hats off to them!"

**Cheryl Millett**, author, *All Guts, All Glory,* Toronto. "If they [dance competitors] eat well, they will never skip a beat as a healthy lifestyle plays a role in winning dancing feet. One and one equals two, nothing else will do!"

**Uzma Naeem,** Calgary. "I like competitive sports and I like competitive dancing. So, I see how people build their skills and put them to work in their dancing as well as to try to make perfect in their passion. It's awesome to see different kinds of people doing this. It's amazing!"

**Maryrose Nakamura,** Newmarket. "When I watch competitive shows like *Dancing with the Stars*, I see how amazing, elegant, and exciting dance can be!"

**Dominic Panacci,** Vaughan, Ontario. "I call them athletes. Their passion, training and competition. You've got to love it!"

**Francesco Pugliese** (sales agent), Toronto. "As a dancer, I regularly follow the TV show *Dancing with the Stars*. I consider it to be a rather instructive and entertaining program and I regard the pairing of celebrities with professional dancers an original and fascinating concept."

**Darren Reid,** Mississauga. "I think it's very entertaining. You can see a lot of beautiful women and the couples are dressed so elegantly and are meshed together dancing."

**Trish Reid,** Mississauga "They must be physically fit so they must be following a special diet that keeps them healthy and slim."

**Raymonde Roy-Pleau,** Comté de Portneuf, Québec. <J'aime dancer et j'aime la danse de bal a mort; c'est si beau, le fun et 170rofessional. J'aurais aimé dancer avec mon épou> *Tanslation*: "I love dancing and love ballroom dancing, it's so beautiful, fun and professional to me. Something I wish I could do with my husband."

**Qasira Shaheen,** Calgary. "I think it's one of the best activities to keep your mind and body in a healthy way and to bring a positive attitude and thoughts while giving you fullness, happiness, softness and humbleness."

**Gerry Shum,** Richmond Hill, Ontario. "It's truly thrilling to watch the couples swirl and float elegantly as if on air to the flowing waltzes, or bounce and turn energetically with lively Latin rhythms. The 'Standards' (the elegant dances) and the 'Latins' (the sensual ones) provide a variety of dances: some are beautiful, some elegant, and some so lively and sexy."

**Arkady Silverman** (university research associate), Toronto. "It's beautiful to see people who have sacrificed their lives for dancing and thrive in it. It really is aspirational and I always come away so much more passion in my own dancing."

**John Stefaniak** (retired forensic photographer), Halifax. "I've enjoyed seeing amateur dancers of limited skill improve in their ability, often to a level that looks quite polished. Such improvements are usually the result of determination, coaching and practice."

**Ashika Theyyil,** Vaughan. "Competitive dance enables confidence. As long as dancers don't solely rely on competition rankings to determine their talent, it's a tremendous opportunity to sharpen technique and for dancers to reach their full potential."

**Silas ("Sie") Tucker**, Newmarket. "Competition dances involve precision with each move perfectly timed with both partners moving in unison as one."

**Daniela Vance**, Port Coquitlam, B.C. "I really enjoy *Dancing with the Stars!* The fast-paced footwork, precision of movement, dazzling costumes, and brilliant partnering of celebrities with professional dancers, to live out their dreams of expressing themselves through dance, makes for great entertainment."

**Susan Vasarhelyi** (breathwork facilitator), Toronto. "I see two entities synchronize their frequencies to produce a fluidic art. To allow them to express how their energies flow between the two of them is truly mesmerizing."

**Issa Veloso** (capacity manager, banking), Aurora. "Competitive dancers encompass superb artistry as seen in the dresses/outfits and the competitors' portrayal of their interpretation of the music as they move through the dance floor."

**Andria W.,** Richmond Hill, Ontario. "I love watching it. It's a combination of things. So, it's beautiful in terms of the mood and their bodies, especially some of the Latin stuff. Just phenomenal. I love the costumes, the theatricality of it."

**Luiza Yavorskay** (hair salon manager), Newmarket. "To dance is to meet the deepest need of our soul. In social and competitive dancing, it is about both social and sexual communication. It's a merging of body and soul. Dancing makes the world of all dancers wider and more voluminous."

# Appendix B: Select list of Canadian Social Dance Academies by Province /Territory and Four Dance Forms

Argentine tango, ballroom/Latin, salsa and square and round dance
(Local government-provided services excluded,
see their seasonal guides for information)

This listing was based on Internet searches and in some cases by phone communication and email. Every effort was made to be accurate and reliable, but there is no guarantee of its authenticity. The list is a guideline only and information may have changed since the book became available. As well, there may be some incorrect or lack of information in the Internet database due to factors beyond the author's control.

## Argentine Tango

### Alberta

- **Ammena Dance Company,** Lethbridge. Lise-Anne Talhami, founder/owner
- **Arthur Murray Dance Centers,** Calgary, Edmonton
- **Beso de Tango Dance Club,** Calgary. Paul Varro, instructor
- **Calgary Milongueros,** Calgary
- **Casa Tango Dance Studio,** Edmonton. Vera Baraz, Daniel Calcines, instructors

- **DC Dance Club,** Calgary. Miro Bartosz, owner/CEO. Carol Violette, instructor
- **Tango Divino,** Edmonton. Vincenzo Renzi, Ida Renzi, instructors **TangoCalgary.com,** Calgary; Foothills County. Leo Sato, lead instructor; Marina Gonzalez, instructor
- **Tango Plus,** Edmonton. Cristina & Vicente, instructors

## British Columbia

- **Alive Tango Victoria,** Victoria. Kelly Henderson, instructor
- **All Vancouver Tango,** Vancouver
- **Argentine Tango Lab,** Vancouver. Gabriel and Sigita, instructors
- **Arthur Murray Dance Centers,** Coquitlam, Vancouver.
- **BC Dance,** Vancouver. Tatiana, instructor
- **Dance Today,** Vancouver. Nina Perez, instructor
- **Dancing for Dessert Ballroom & Latin Dance Studio,** Langley. Magda Rudzik, studio director. Andrew McIntosh, dance director, Trevor Bunt, Claire Houghton, instructors
- **La Tangueria Esposito,** Vancouver. Clarry & Elizbeth, instructors
- **Magic Tango,** Vancouver. Tatiana Balashova, instructor
- **Portal A Tango,** Abbotsford, Chilliwack, Richmond, Surrey
- **Sharon Sebo Dance/Tango Kelowna,** Kelowna. Sharon Sebo, instructor
- **Steven Joanna Tango,** Vancouver. Steven & Joanna, instructors
- **Strictly Tango,** Vancouver, Nadia Tavakoli, instructor
- **Sueños Tango,** Cranbrook. Sharlene Harden & Dennis, instructors
- **Tango Vancouver.com,** Vancouver. Susana Domingues, instructor
- **Tangobug.com.** Langley. Bobbi Lusic, Patricia Lusic, instructors
- **The Tango Studio,** Vancouver. Santiago Yanez, Deborah Lynne, instructors; Georgi Genchev, practica host
- **Vancouver Tango Milonguero,** Vancouver. Semiral, Pimon, Jud, hosts
- **World Dance Company,** Burnaby. Ekaterina Mitchtchenko, Roland Mitchtchenko, instructors

## Manitoba

- **Patricia's Dance Studio**, Winnipeg
- **Shirley's Dance Studio**, Winnipeg. Shirley Caron, instructor
- **Tango Salon Winnipeg**, Winnipeg. Alberto and Fernanda, instructors
- **University of Manitoba's Active Learning Centre, Winnipeg, Horace Luong, instructor**
- **Winnipeg Tango Projects**, Winnipeg. Philbert Furere, Irina Blinova, instructors
- **Winnipeg Argentine Tango Community**, Winnipeg

## New Brunswick, Newfoundland & Labrador

- **Jill Dreaddy DanceCo.,** St John's, Conception Bay S., Jill Dreaddy principal

## Nova Scotia

- **Halifax Tango Community**, Halifax
- **LINDance**, Bridgewater, Liverpool, Lunenberg, Mahone Bay. Heidrun T. Lind, instructor
- **You, Two, Can Tango**, Halifax. Martina Sommer, Lorne Buick, principals
- **Tangonova**, Halifax. Margaret Spore, instructor.
- **Tea & Tango**, Halifax. Lorne Buick, Martina Sommer, Jackie Webster, hosts

## Ontario

- **Access Ballroom**, Toronto. Monica P. Bautistia, instructor
- **Adam Czub's School of Dance,** Toronto
- **Anna's Dance Centre,** Toronto
- **Argentine Tango Toronto El Abrazo,** Toronto. Andy Kamienski, director
- **Argentine Tango Markham/Stouffville** (public group), Markham
- **Art Gallery of Ontario @Walker Court,** Toronto

- **Artistica Ballroom Dance Studio Inc.,** Aurora. Kelly Stacey, Patrick Derry, co-owners/instructors; Anastasia Trutneva, instructor
- **Arthur Murray Dance Centers,** Ajax, Toronto (Etobicoke, North York, "Yorkville,"), Oakville, Ottawa, Vaughan, Waterloo
- **Ballroom Class,** Guelph. Michelle Ariss, owner
- **Belmonte Tango Academy,** Toronto. Roxana Belmonte, Fabian Belmonte, instructors
- **Argentine Tango Toronto,** Toronto. Bulent Karabagli, Lina Chan, instructors
- **Chrisa Assis/Steve Yee,** Toronto
- **City Dance Corps,** Toronto. Jerome Jean-Gilles, Estelle Nichol, Tina Nico, co-founders/directors; Madison Burgess, youth program director
- **Club Milonga,** Toronto. Doug Gilbertson, president.
- **Dance Fire Studio,** Richmond Hill. Viara Vranska, principal
- **Dance Time,** Toronto. Halina Bodnar, instructor
- **Dance With Me Toronto,** Toronto, Markham & Richmond Hill. Egor Belashow, founder
- **El Studio Tango,** London. Milena Todorovic, Ross Todorovic, instructors.
- **GTA Tango,** Hamilton. Zubair S., director
- **Gary/Sahori Dafoe,** Toronto
- **Grand Dance Studio,** Vaughan. Angelika Kasparova, Anna Pelypenko, Vlad Vinogradsky, Tatyana Vovkokhat, instructors
- **Joy of Dance Centre,** Toronto. Joyce Audrey Jones, founder. Linda Walsh, instructor
- **Latin Energy Dance Studio,** Mississauga. Vanesa Stay, principal
- **Learn to Dance,** Brampton. Susie Roach, instructor
- **Let Us Dance,** Toronto. Sergei Filushkin, instructor
- **Melina Martinez Andretto,** Toronto
- **Miguel Y/Michelle Coppini,** Cambridge, Guelph, Kitchener, and Waterloo. Miguel Coppini, Michel Coppini, instructors
- **Milonga Maleva,** Toronto
- **N2Tango,** Toronto. Nina, Nick, instructors
- **Olympic Stars Dance Academy,** Vaughan. Aruna Bizokas, owner/instructor.
- **Paradise Tango,** Toronto
- **PointeTango,** London. Alex and Erin, instructors

- **Queen's University Salsa Club,** Kingston
- **Rhythm & Motion Dance Studio,** Toronto. Elizabeth Sadlowska, director. Sergei Filushkin, Tarek Marroushi, Linda Smith, instructors
- **Ruben Bustamente,** Toronto.
- **Sandra Maria Rocha,** Toronto. instructor
- **Siempre Tango,** Ottawa
- **Star Dance Centre**, Toronto
- **Tango Academy,** Windsor
- **Tango Soul,** Toronto. Bryant Lopez, Faye Lavin, instructors
- **The Ballroom Class,** Guelph. Michelle Ariss, owner
- **Toronto Dance Spot,** Toronto.
- **Toronto Tango Club,** Toronto
- **Toronto Tango Experience,** German Ballejo, Micaela Colleen Barrett, Albert Ramos Cordero, Carlitos Espinoza, Magdalena Gutierrez Noelia Hurtado, Eleonora Kalganova,
- **University of Toronto Argentine Tango Club,** Toronto

## Prince Edward Island

No Argentine tango dance studios identified.

## Québec

- **Arthur Murray Dance Studio,** Dollard-des-Ormeaux, Laval, Montréal, Québec City
- **Concordia University Recreation,** Montréal
- **Dance Conmigo,** Montréal. Alain Guillot, Cheryl Williams, instructors
- **Studio Tango Montréal,** Montréal

## Saskatchewan

- **Argentine Tango Saskatoon**, Saskatoon.
- **Danza Morena Latin Dance Academy**, Saskatoon. Carmen Gonza, principal. Elaine Masich, Michael Mondor, Penny Schafer, instructors

# Ballroom/Latin

## Alberta

- **ACDA Dance Studio**, Calgary, Grand Prairie, Red Deer. Dale Toszak, instructor
- **Alberta Ballroom Company**, Bryan Senn, Lisa Senn, co-owners. Ryan Anderson, Christine Mooney, Bryan Senn, instructors
- **Alberta DanceSport**, Calgary. Eric Caty, Kelly Lanan, instructors
- **Ammena Dance Company**, Lethbridge. Lise-Anne Talhami, founder/owner
- **Arthur Murray Dance Studio**, Edmonton, Calgary.
- **Ballroom and Country Dance Studio**, Calgary. Thu Luu, owner/instructor. Jesse Yap, instructor
- **DC Dance Club**, Calgary. Miro Bartosz, owner/CEO. Angela K., instructor
- **Dance on Cloud Nine**, Edmonton. Steve Natran, instructor
- **Dancing Til Dawn**, Calgary. Dawn Erath, instructor
- **Elite Dance Studio**, Edmonton. Katie Cameron, Jim Deglau, Kevin & Sheena, Dominic Lacroix, Grace Lau, Elena Modzolevska, Elijah Ocean, Delphine Romaire, Anton Szabo, instructors
- **Everyone's Ballroom Dance Association**, Edmonton. Frank Colpitts, Bob Mellor, Peter Van Hogezand, Viki Van Hogezand, Dorothea Thielmann, executive members
- **Foot Notes Dance Studio**, Edmonton
- **Levita Dance Studio**, Calgary. Dmitry Levita, Aleksandra Antonova, instructors
- **Medicine Hat Ballroom Dance Club**, Redcliff
- **Panko Dance Ballroom & DanceSport Studio**, Edmonton. Devon Panko, head instructor
- **Rhythms of Dance**, Calgary. Cindy Tymko, Richard Tymko, instructors
- **Shok Dance**, Calgary
- **Studio G Dance Art**, Edmonton
- **The Calgary Dance Club**, Calgary TJ Al-Himyary, president
- **University of Alberta Dance Club**, Edmonton.

## British Columbia

- **Arthur Murray Dance Studio,** Vancouver, White Rock, Coquitlam
- **Bez Arts Hub**, Langley
- **Broadway Ballroom**, Vancouver. Michelle Peng, owner/instructor
- **Corta Jaca Dance,** Bowser. Andy Mundy, Maureen Mundy, principals and instructors
- **D Boyerdance,** Vancouver. Dominic Boyer, instructor
- **Dale Neale Dance,** Vancouver. Dale Neale, instructor
- **Dance Discovery Social Dance School,** Kamloops. Teresa Carroll, instructor
- **Dance Town**, Vancouver. Maggie Denise Bretton, instructor.
- **Dance with Me Studio** New Westminster. Janice Stevens, owner
- **Dancing for Dessert Ballroom & Latin Dance Studio,** Langley. Magda Rudzik, studio director. Andrew McIntosh, dance director, Trevor Bunt, Claire Houghton, instructors
- **Delta Dance,** Delta, Surrey. George Pytlik, Wendy Pytlik, co-owners/instructors
- **Dominic Boyer Ballroom Dance,** Vancouver. Dominic Boyer, instructor
- **E & R Ballroom Dance,** Victoria. Elizabeth Smailes, Ron Smailes, co-owners/ instructors
- **Kyryl Dance**, Richmond. Kyryl Dudchenko, instructor.
- **Crystal Ballroom**, Vancouver. Peter Chen, Angel Chu, Tony Fung, Faye Hung, Sarah Liang, Mark Ma, Dimitri Milkulich, Neli Petkova, Kessa Wills, Zillion Wong, Laurie Xie and Linda Zhang, instructors
- **Dream Maker Dance Studio**, Victoria. Taneya, instructor
- **Imperial Ballroom**, Richmond. Crystal Li, Han Ly, instructors
- **JC Dance Co.**, Vancouver. Clara Shih Marasigan, Joel Marasigan, co-owners/instructors
- **Kelowna Ballroom,** Kelowna. Chris Thorburn, instructor
- **Mr Dance @Vancouver Alpen Club,** Michael, co-creator; Elsie, Frankie, Ken, Steven, instructors
- **Sam's Dance,** Vancouver. Patricia Hardin, founder, Simone Fragoso, Hugo Okajima, instructors
- **Sharon Sebo Dance/Tango Kelowna,** Kelowna. Sharon Sebo, instructor

- **TG DanceSport**, Vancouver. Tony & Gloria, instructors
- **The Grand Ballroom**, Vancouver. Andy Wong, Wendy Wong, co-owners/instructors
- **University of British Columbia Dance Club**, Vancouver. Patricia Melgar, president; Brian Andrew, Phoebe Lin, Wendy Leung, Joshua Pablo, Hala-Murad Ch, Wendy Song, Christine Trites, Nicholas Zheng, executive members
- **University of Victoria (UVIC) Ballroom, Latin and Swing Club**, Victoria. Will Beckett, president. Chris Friedrich, Guiseppe Travaglini, Jo Spry, executive members
- **Vancouver Academy of Ballroom Dance**, Vancouver. Dale Neale, director; Bea Rhodes, instructor
- **Victory Dance Club**, Vancouver. Vlad, Sarah, instructors
- **Yasel DanceSport Academy**, Vancouver. Viktor Yasel, Irina Prodan,
- Instructors
- **World Dance Company**, Burnaby. Ekaterina Mitchtchenko, Roland Mitchtchenko, instructors

## Manitoba

- **Shirley's Dance Studio**, Winnipeg.: Shirley Caron, owner/instructor
- **Ted Motyka Dance Studio**, Winnipeg. Ted Motyka, instructor
- **VS Dance Club**, Vancouver.

## New Brunswick

- **Headpond Dance Studio**, Fredericton.
- **Aurele Belliveau School of Dance**, Moncton
- **KV Ballroom Dancing, Rothesay**, Quispamsis.
- **Mary Cain Dance**, Moncton. Mary Cain, principal & instructor.

## Newfoundland and Labrador

- **Jill Dreaddy Danceco**, St. John's, Conception Bay South. Jill Dreaddy, principal and artistic director. Adele Walsh, Abby Rowe, instructors; Julia Antle, Brooke Boland, Deirdre Hartley, Lola Power, Emily Smith, Maisy Sullivan, Anna Williams, teaching assistants

- **MUN (Memorial University of Newfoundland) Ballroom & Latin Dance Club,** St. John's. Laura Dawson, club president. Shaelynn Barry, Tyra Dawe, Sara Hawkins, Alyson Judd, Megan Reid, Shramana Sarkar, executive members; Christine Greening, Jim Russell, Andrea Scherle, instructors

## Nova Scotia

- **Ballroom with Brenton,** Bedford. Brenton Mitchell, owner/instructor
- **Concept Creative Dance Center,** Sydney. Chris Mkandawire, executive director. Kara Raoul, instructor
- **Dancing with Michel & Company,** Halifax. Michel Dubé, owner. Trena Graham, Stacie Kelly, Jan Ainslie, Elisa Wong, instructors
- **Edgett Dance & Wellness,** Halifax. Brenton Mitchell, owner/instructor. Barb Child, Ian Crewe, Janet Edgett, Janet Hartman, Nadia Kisaleva, Kathy Murphy, instructors

## Ontario

- **Abanico Dance,** Toronto. Karen Lee Rodriguez-Chaba, owner/director; Alessandra Amaro, studio manager; Ole Olavide, instructor
- **Abby Mina,** Toronto.
- **Academy of Ballroom Dance,** Sudbury. Carla Cox, Peter Cox, instructors
- **Access Ballroom Studio,** Toronto. Monica P. Bautistia, instructor
- **Arthur Murray Dance Centers,** Ajax, Toronto (Etobicoke, North York, "Yorkville,"), Oakville, Ottawa, Vaughan
- **Art in Motion Dance Studio,** Brantford.
- **Artur Adamski,** Toronto
- **Alexsandra Plaza,** Toronto
- **All Star Dance Studio,** Hamilton. Marie Zimmer, principal
- **Andras Ballroom Academy,** Vaughan. Andras I. Urniezius, instructor
- **Anna's Dance Centre,** Toronto
- **Arthur Murray Dance Centers,** Ajax, Mississauga, Oakville, Ottawa, Richmond Hill, Stoney Creek, Toronto (Etobicoke, North York, "Yorkville,"), Vaughan, Waterloo
- **Art in Motion Dance Studio,** Brantford.

- **Artur Adamski,** Toronto
- **Ballroom and Latin Dance Studio in Niagara,** Thorold. Chamari, Dan Matkowski, instructors
- **Ballroom and Latin Dancing with Bob and Mary,** London. Bob Rowswell, Mary Rowswell, instructors
- **Ballroom At Its Best,** Windsor. Claire Hansen, Richard Tonizzo, Amy Nabbout, instructors
- **Ballroom Basics,** Lincoln. Herb Schoss, instructor
- **Ballroom Blitz Dance Studio,** London.
- **Ballroom Class,** Guelph. Michelle Ariss, owner
- **Ballroom Dance Studies,** Richmond Hill, Markham and Toronto. Vincent Luk, principal
- **Ballroom Dance Studios,** Sudbury. Catherine Clark, Dennis Harasymchuk, Colette Lance, Dale Mansfield, Linda Smania, instructors
- **Ballroom Health Dance Studio,** Halton Hills
- **Ballroom in Bloom,** London. Rob Campbell, instructor
- **Ballroom on Bayview,** Toronto. Oleg Yedlin, founder/director. Linda Marsella, Christine Moszynski, Steven James. instructors
- **Blueheel Dance Studio,** Mississauga. Bee Songvilay, Caroline Augustin, founders
- **Bob and Mary Rowswell,** London.
- **Boléo Latin & Ballroom Dance Studio,** Oakville.
- **BOW Dance with Vlad.** Burlington. Vladimir Chernyshov, instructor
- **CM Cha Cha Cha Dance Studio,** Markham. Carlo Tran, Monica Tran, co-owners/instructors Jitka Bouma.
- **Chance Dance Centre,** Newmarket. Sergey Muretov, instructor
- **Ciao Bella Dance Studio,** Vaughan
- **Club Paradise 2 Dance Studio,** Vaughan. Stefano Corapi, Margaret Ottaviani, instructors
- **Come Dancing!** Mississauga.
- **Dance2Impress,** Toronto. Christopher Sochnacki, instructor
- **Dance DNA,** Vaughan. Anna Smodlev, Nikolay Smodlev, co-owners; Tikhostoup Catherine, Evgeniya Gorobets, Anna Kaplii, Irina Khanova, Alex Maslanka, Olga Nor-Arevian, Michael Rubezin, Kamil Studenny, Timchenko Victor, instructors
- **DanceLife Studios,** Toronto. Zilvinas Vaidila, Aira Vaidila, co-founders. Hugo Vaidila, Nino Langella, Richard Lifshitz, Alex Maslanka,

Laura Robinson, Andra Vaidilaite, Maurizio Vescovo, Alex Maslanka, instructors
- **DanceLife X Centre,** Toronto.
- **DanceScape Dance Club & Studio,** Burlington. Robert Tang, Beverley Cayton-Tang, co-owners/instructors
- **DanceTown Inc.,** Ottawa. Dane Harris, owner. Murray Carter, Chris Drumm, Lorna Jackle, Maxim Kazakoff, Kamila Lichvárová, Rick Ruggles, Matt Salama, Shanna Salama, Dmytro Startsev, Melanie Strickland. instructors
- **Dance Art Studio,** Richmond Hill. Cristina Amalia Dina, owner/instructor
- **Dance Club Blue Silver,** Richmond Hill. Phil Lee, Patricia Goh, instructors
- **Dance Fire Studio,** Richmond Hill. Viara Vranska, owner/principal
- **Dance Spirit Club, Toronto.** Konstantin Antonov, owner/instructor
- **Dance to the Rhythm Studio,** Mississauga. Rosalie Francisco, owner/choreographer. Allan Torres, instructor
- **Danceline Studios**, Hamilton
- **Dance Now,** Toronto
- **Dance Spirit Club,** Toronto. Konstantin Antonov, owner/instructor
- **Dance Time**, Toronto. Halina Bodnar, instructor
- **Dance Together Project,** Toronto. Katya Kuznetsova, owner/instructor
- **Dance Town Inc.,** Ottawa. Dane Harris, owner
- **Dance with Me Toronto,** Toronto, Markham & Richmond Hill. Egor Belashov, principal and instructor
- **Dance with Gus, London.** Gus Braun, instructor
- **Dance with Sharon,** Toronto. Sharon Cai, instructor
- **Dance with TLC,** Ottawa. TL & Chris Rader, instructors
- **Dance with Us Ottawa,** Ottawa. Yuriy Shelkovvy, Oksana Shelkovvy, Ilya Maletin, Remy Bourquin, instructors
- **Dance Hollingsworth,** Waterloo. Roger Hollingsworth, Moira Hollingsworth, instructors
- **Dance Masters,** Vaughan. Agita Baranovska, founder. Maria, Daniil, Kevin and Polina
- **Dance National Academy,** Vaughan. Nikolay Smodlev, Anna Smodlev, co-owners. Tikhostoup Catherine, Anna Kaplii, Irina

Khanova, Evgeniya Gorobets, Olga Nor-Arevian, Alex Maslanka, Michael Rubezin, Kamil Studenny, Victor Timchenko, instructors
- **Dance Stream Studio,** Vaughan. Sergey Shvaitser, owner/artistic director. Elena Shvaitser, instructor
- **Dancin' Di's,** Kitchener. Diana Greenlay, instructor
- **Dancingland Dance Studio,** East Gwillimbury, Toronto, Vaughan. George Kastulin, owner/principal instructor
- **DanSteps,** Hamilton, Oakville and Toronto. Dan Lee, principal
- **Danse Avec Moi,** Milton. Jean-Guy Bernard, founder/president
- **Dancing with Steve Nelson,** Toronto
- **EdmundsTowers School of Dance,** Windsor.
- **Enamorarse Dance,** Richmond Hill.
- **5678 Dance Studio,** Kingston.
- **Flying Dance Community,** Guelph. Nicholas Muthui Kaburia, director
- **Fred Astaire Dance Studios,** Hamilton, Kitchener, London, Oakville, Ottawa
- **GTA Dance School,** Toronto. Alexandre Chalkevich, instructor
- **Gordon Fong,** Toronto, Mississauga.
- **Grand Dance Studio,** Vaughan. Angelika Kasparova, Anna Pelypenko, Vlad Vinogradsky, Tatyana Vovkokhat, instructors
- **HH Dance Studio,** Markham. Henry Yang, Helen Hu, owners/principals
- **Join the Dance (Canada),** Pickering. Ilsa Abraham, principal
- **Joli's Dance Studio,** Welland. Jolan Sniegocki, owner/director founder
- **Joy of Dance Centre,** Toronto. Joyce Audrey Jones, founder. Olé Burlay, Danielito Guajardo, Nicole Heinecke, Steven James, Milena Kolarova, Annie Lebedeva, Rebecca Lewis, Linda Marsella, Arpad Raymon, Mark Read, Lisa Scarfo, Julia Vokhmina, instructors
- **Judy's School of Dance,** Stratford. Judy Waymouth, owner/operator
- **L'Ambiance Dance Centre,** Toronto, Al Wahab, instructor
- **Lakeside Dance Studio,** Innisfil. Ashley & Adam, instructors
- **Larry Hall,** Toronto
- **Learn to Dance,** Brampton. Susie Roach, studio manager
- **Let's Dance London,** London. Julia Cassis, instructor
- **Let Us Dance,** Toronto. Sergei Filushkin, instructor
- **Love to Dance,** Toronto

- **Lucille's Ball Dance Club,** Burlington. Lucy, owner/instructor
- **Mandy's Dance,** Mississauga. Mandy Epprecht, principal & instructor
- **McMaster Centre for Dance,** Hamilton. Dave Wilson, artistic director
- **Michael's Dance Floor,** St. Thomas. Michael Murphy, instructor
- **National Ballroom Academy,** Toronto. Glen Michael, founder/president. Melina Xu, Mark Shpuntov, Ronen Cherniavski, instructors
- **Niagara Falls Dance,** St Catharines, Niagara-on-the-Lake, Fort Erie, Port Colborne, Welland. Amaury VT, owner
- **Olé to Dance,** Oakville, Dania Marin, owner/principal
- **Olympic Stars Dance Academy,** Vaughan. Aruna Bizokas, owner/instructor. Konstantin Antonov, Igor Fylymonchyk, Alon Gilin, Serghei Kirichenko, Stanislav Kochergin, Marius Kriukelis, Inna, Jen Lee, Anna Pelypenko, Sergei Pogonet, Svetlana Sokolski, Inessa Strelnikova, Maryna Turturika, Tatiana Vainer, instructors
- **Ottawa Dance Sport Studio,** Ottawa. Milla Sekret, owner
- **Passion for Dance,** London. Pamela Forbes, owner/instructor
- **Rainbow Rhythm Ballroom Dance Group,** Kitchener-Waterloo. James Hobson, Julie Hobson, instructors
- **Rhythm & Motion,** Toronto. Elizabeth Sadowska, director. Yurate Banis, Alexander De Ronov, Steve Murgatroyd, instructors
- **Richard J. Thibault,** Toronto
- **Salchata Dance Academy,** Toronto, Oriana and Sam
- **Shall We Dance Studio,** Toronto. Maria Golovanevski, director/founder; Masha Iluykhina, Ivan Levedev, Val Mirosh, Yvan Piwovarov, instructors
- **Silver Steps Dance Studio,** Arnprior. Yasemin Gumus, owner/instructor
- **Simply Ballroom and Latin Studios,** Burlington
- **SlavaTalent Ballroom Dance Studio,** Ottawa. Veycheslav Tudorovsky, Stephanie Tudorovsky, instructors
- **Slyde Ballroom and DanceSport,** London, Sarnia
- **Star Dance Centre,** Toronto. Fiona Su, owner/CEO
- **Star Potential Studios,** Toronto. Ellen Annor-Adjel, owner. Vlacheslav Chizhik, instructor
- **Steve Miller Dance,** southern Ontario
- **Stilian Kostov Dance Studio,** Toronto. Stilian Kostov, founder & instructor

- **Szwec School of Dance,** Hamilton, Marilyn Szwec, director
- **The Ballroom Dance Studio,** Hamilton. Jesse V., owner/instructor
- **The Continental Dance Club,** Mississauga. Brian R. Torner, owner. Sylvain Cardinal, Denis Tremblay, instructors
- **The DanceLive X Centre,** Toronto
- **The Dance Centre,** Toronto. Al Wahab, instructor
- **The London Ballroom Dance Club Inc.**, London. Lawrence McKenzie, president. Valery Didinchuk, Andrew Habib, Marie-Thérèse Habib, Cathy Penalagan, Beth Maybury, executive members; see https://www.londonballroomdanceclub.ca/ for instructors.
- **30-Up Club,** Toronto. Marjorie White, president. Tom Berend, Carol DiMillo, Peter Lee, Cathy Primeau, Joanne Pritchard, Vivianne Schinkel, Michelle Strom, Peter van Tol, Justin White, directors; Ruth Dyson, standing committee member; see Home (30-up.com) for instructors.
- **Toronto Ballroom Academy, Toronto.** Alexandre Chalkevich, instructor
- **Toronto Dance Professionals,** Toronto. Deniz Karakulak, principal
- **Vallerandance,** Shakespeare. Melody Vallerand, François Vallerand, owners & instructors
- **Toronto Dance Professionals,** Toronto. Deniz Karakulak, owner
- **U of T Ballroom Latin Dance Club, Toronto.** Maxim Kazakoff, Myriam Savaria, instructors. Louise Wang, president. Benjamin Piette, executive member
- **Waterloo Dance,** Kitchener. Vladyslav Komelkov, Alexandra Sevastianova, instructors
- **West-Way Dance Club (The),** Toronto. Mary Fulton, Brian Kearney, Collette Lapointe-Kearney, Nenad Miric, Eva Novak, Danny Sheehan, Corinne Tripsansky, Grace Zhang, directors
- **Yourweddingdance.ca,** Toronto. George Kastulin, owner/instructor

# Prince Edward Island

- **DownStreet Dance Studio**, Charlottetown
- **Ballroom Barn Dance Studio**, Hunter River

## Québéc

- **Academie de Danse Fanny Godin**, Québec
- **Alex Sharov Dance Studio**, Hudson. Alex Sharov, instructor
- **Arthur Murray Dance Centers**, Dollard-des-Ormeaux, Laval, Montréal, Québec City
- **Centre Ballroom DanceSport**, Montréal,
- **Centre de Danse Jacques Duval**, Québec City
- **Concordia University Recreation & Athletics**, Montréal
- **Confidanse**, Montréal
- **Dance Conmigo**, Montréal. Alain Guillot, Cheryl Williams, instructors
- **DuoDanse Dance School Ballroom**, L'Île-Bizard. Serge Fortier, instructor
- **École de Danse Grenier**, Varennes. Andrée Grenier, Manon Grenier, co-owners/instructors
- **École de Danse Sportive 'Quartier Latin'**, Montréal
- **FollowMaxFomin**, Montréal. Max Fomin, principal
- **Juste Danse Ballroom**, Montréal
- **Julie Bergeron Danse Sociale**, Laval. Julie Bergeron, principal
- **Lebedev Dance**, Montréal. Anton Lebedev, owner
- **Studio 2720 Canada**, Montréal. Mathieu Casavant, director
- **Studio Danza, Pierrefonds**. Danny Arbour, Justine Rainville, co-founders/directors
- **Studio Juste Danse**, Montréal. Allyson Kassie, owner
- **Studio Musique et Danse**, Montréal.
- **TS Dance Studio**, Westmount. Tony Santana, instructor
- **Universal Dance Studio**, Montréal. Maria, Vanessa, instructors
- **Westmount Dance Studio**, Montréal

## Saskatchewan

- **Dance Class Saskatoon**, Saskatoon
- **Dance Dynamics**, Saskatoon. Herb Clarke, manager. Holly Horel, Greg Schneider, instructors
- **Dance on Cloud Nine**, Stony Plain, Fort Saskatchewan. Steve Natran, instructor.

# Salsa

## Alberta

- **Alberta DanceSport,** Calgary. Eric Caty, Kelly Lanan, directors. David Joseph, Olya Joseph, instructors
- **Ammena Dance Company,** Lethbridge, Lise-Anne Talhami, founder/owner
- **DC Dance Club,** Calgary. Miro Bartosz, owner/CEO. Edward C., Angela K. instructors
- **Etown Salsa Latin Dance Studios,** Edmonton. Alejandro Rojas, Carlos Ruedas Velasco, instructors; Ana Rojas, Tanya Murray, assistants
- **Fiesta Cubana Dance School,** Edmonton.
- **Foot Notes Dance Studio,** Edmonton
- **Havana Cuban Dance Studio,** Calgary. Marcos Ravelo, owner/director/instructor; Mandie Black, studio manager; Nathalie Berard, Katreena Cardenas, Steph Erlendson, Alex Kos, Natalie Melara, Luis Valdes, instructors
- **Latin Corner Dance Studio,** Calgary
- **Mambo Productions Latin Dance School**, Calgary. David, director; Alex, Elena, Lucy, Melvin, instructors
- **More Salsa,** Calgary. Max Posadas, Melissa Posadas, instructors
- **Rhythms Dance Studio,** Edmonton. Chad, instructor
- **Salsaddiction Dance Company,** Edmonton. Usukuma Ekuere, founder/instructor
- **Shok Dance,** Calgary.
- **Unleashed Dance Company,** Calgary. Angela Mulrooney, founder/lead choreographer; Erin Prosser, owner/instructor. Laura Distefano, Fiorella Giovannetti, Sheena Lambert, Lev Oshchepkov, Tatiana Oshchepkova, Danielle Sheehan, instructors

## British Columbia

- **Adagé Studio**, Duncan.
- **BC Dance Co.,** Vancouver. Nestor, instructor.
- **Baila! Dance Toda**, Vancouver. Nina Perez, instructor

- **Baza Dance Studios**, Vancouver. Kristal Barbaza, Wayne Barbaza, co-directors/owners/instructors; Arely Santana, Celina Villarroel Whiting, instructors
- **Bravo Dance Company**, Vancouver, Burnaby. Alfonso Caldera, instructor
- **D2 Dance Studio**, Vancouver. Patrick Moriarty and Scarlet Moriarty, instructors
- **Dance4U**, Vancouver. Corey Solomon, Samia Massoud, Jessica Sage, instructors
- **Dance Dojo**, Vancouver. Robin Campbell, Cody Campbell, co-founders; Patrick Moriarity, Scarlet Moriarity, instructors
- **Dancing for Dessert Ballroom & Latin Dance Studio**, Langley. Magda Rudzik, studio director. Andrew McIntosh, dance director, Trevor Bunt, Claire Houghton, instructors
- **Dance With Me Studio**, New Westminster. Janice Stevens, owner
- **Dominic Boyer Ballroom Dance**, Vancouver. Dominic Boyer, instructor
- **Hot Salsa Dance Zone**, Coquitlam, Port Coquitlam, Port Moody, Surrey. Alberto Gonzalez, Teresa Szefler, instructors
- **Kelowna Ballroom**, Kelowna. Chris Thorburn, instructor
- **Latin Beat Dance Club**, Vancouver. Susi Haemmerle, owner/instructor
- **Latin Dance Canada.com**, Victoria. Ronald Martinez, director/mentor/instructor
- **Salsastudio Vancouver**, Vancouver. Roger Chen, head instructor/director
- **Salsa Caliente!** Victoria. Christina Morrison, director
- **Salsa Moderna Dance Studio**, Victoria. Bernard Henin, instructor
- **Salsa Vancouver**, Patrick Moriarity, Scarlet Moriarity, instructors
- **Sam's Dance**, Vancouver. Patricia Hardin, founder
- **Sharon Sebo Dance/Tango Kelowna**, Kelowna. Sharon Sebo, instructor
- **Vancouver Latin Fever (VLF)**, Vancouver. VLF hosts guest instructors
- **World Dance Company**, Burnaby. Diego Sanchez, instructor

## Manitoba

- **Dance World,** Winnipeg. Regan Hirose, Harold Rancano, founders. Jedi Baker, Bennett Murphy, Schaeffer Murphy, Amelie, Kelly, Lorna, Mary, Melanie, Suzie, Thomas, instructors
- **Salsa Explosion Dance Co.**, Winnipeg. Ana Karen Lopez, Leonardo Lopez, directors
- **Ted Motyka Dance Studio,** Winnipeg. Ted Motyka, instructor

## New Brunswick

- **Belliveau Aurele School of Dance**, Moncton
- **Headpond Dance Studio**, Fredericton
- **Mary Cain Dance**, Moncton. Mary Cain, principal & instructor.

## Newfoundland & Labrador

- **Bailamos St John's**, St. John's.
- **Dance Studio West**, Corner Brook
- **MUN (Memorial University of Newfoundland) Ballroom & Latin Dance Club**, St. John's. Christine Greening, Jim Russell, Andrea Scherle, instructors. Laura Dawson, club president. Shaelynn Barry, Tyra Dawe, Sara Hawkins, Alyson Judd, Megan Reid, Shramana Sarkar, executive members
- **Salsa in St John's**, St. John's

## Nova Scotia

- **Concept Creative Dance Company,** Sydney. Chris Mkandawire, executive director. Baillie Ferguson, instructor
- **Haliente Dance Studio,** Halifax. Moses Diallo, owner/director; Amanda Ivey, operations director. Yuyu, instructor
- **Trena's Studio**, Bedford. Trema Graham, owner & instructor
- **Halifax Salseros,** Halifax. Danny Godfrey, Cindy Davis, instructors.

## Ontario

- **Abanico Dance**, Toronto. Karen Lee Rodriguez-Chaba, owner/director; Alessandra Amaro, studio manager. Maya Charley, Andrew Gray, Yordan Guttiérrez, instructors
- **Araguacu Latin Dance Company**, Toronto. Kimberly Ramos, Geovanny Ricardo, co-founders/co-directors
- **Abby Mina,** Toronto.
- **Access Ballroom Studio**, Toronto. Monica P. Bautistia, instructor
- **AfroLatino Dance Company,** Toronto. Albena de Assis, director/instructor. Karen Bender, Karen Green, Miranda Liverpool, Sax Salsera, Anny Yudina, instructors
- **Alexsandra Plaza,** Toronto
- **Anna's Dance Centre,** Toronto
- **Araguacu Latin Dance Company,** Toronto.
- **Arthur Murray Dance Centers,** Ajax, Mississauga, Toronto (Etobicoke, North York, "Yorkville,"), Oakville, Ottawa, Richmond Hill, Stoney Creek, Vaughan, Waterloo
- **Artur Adamski,** Toronto
- **Azucar! Latin Dance Company,** Ottawa. Ana Gherasim, owner/founder. Talek Cameron, Paige Reno, Stephane Bernadel, instructors
- **Ballroom Class,** Guelph. Michelle Ariss, owner
- **Ballroom Dance Studios,** Sudbury. Catherine Clark, Dennis Harasymchuk, Colette Lance, Dale Mansfield, Linda Smania, instructors
- **CM Cha Cha Cha Dance Studio,** Markham. Carlo Tran, Monica Tran, Jitka Bouma, instructors
- **Carlos & Sofia Show Dance,** Toronto, Carlos Zapata, Sofia Skvirsky, co-owners/principals
- **City Dance Corps,** Toronto. Jerome Jean-Gilles, Estelle Nico, Tina Nico, co-founders/directors; Madison Burgess, youth program director
- **Dan Steps,** Hamilton, Oakville, Toronto. Dan Lee, instructor
- **DanceTown Inc.,** Ottawa. Dane Harris, owner. Murray Carter, Chris Drumm, Lorna Jackle, Maxim Kazakoff, Kamila Lichvárová, Rick Ruggles, Matt Salama, Shanna Salama, Dmytro Startsev, Melanie Strickland. instructors
- **Dance To Live Studio,** Toronto. Paula Videla-Rodriguez, Jose Rodriguez, co/owners/instructors

- **Dance Art Studio,** Richmond Hill. Cristina Amalia Dina, instructor
- **Dance ConneXion,** Toronto. Tania Wong, artistic director
- **DanceScape Dance Club & Studio,** Burlington. Robert Tang, Beverley Cayton-Tang, co-owners/instructors
- **Dance Time,** Toronto. Halina Bodnar, instructor
- **Dance to Live Studio,** Toronto. Paula Videla-Rodriguez, José Rodriguez, co-founders/co-directors
- **Dance with Gus, London.** Gus Braun, instructor
- **Dance with Me!** Cobourg. Gabia Antony, instructor
- **Dance with Me Toronto,** Toronto, Markham & Richmond Hill. Egor Belashov, principal and instructor
- **Dance with Sharon,** Toronto. Sharon Cai, instructor
- **Dance Fire Studio,** Richmond Hill. Viara Vranska, principal
- **Dance Social Toronto Events,** Toronto. Frank Bishun, owner
- **Dancingland Dance Studio,** East Gwillimbury, Toronto, Vaughan. George Kastulin, owner/principal instructor
- **Dancing Thru Life,** Burlington. Peter Djakovic, instructor
- **DY Dance,** Toronto. Dora Yaneva, instructor
- **Everybuddy Dance Studios,** Guelph.
- **Flying Dance Community,** Guelph. Nicholas Muthui Kaburia, director
- **Fred Astaire Franchised Dance Studios,** Hamilton, Kitchener, London, Oakville, Ottawa
- **Grand Dance Studio,** Vaughan. Angelika Kasparova, Anna Pelypenko, Vlad Vinogradsky, Tatyana Vovkokhat, instructors
- **iFreeStyle.ca,** Toronto. Caryl Cuizon, Angus Dirnbeck, Mo Kobrosli, senior instructors. Joey Lopez, Andre Marto, Maria Linares, instructors
- **isalsaInToronto,** Toronto. Nixon Nguyen, instructor
- **Joli's Dance Studio,** Welland. Jolan Sniegocki, owner/director
- **Latin Energy Dance Studio,** Mississauga. Vanesa Stay, principal
- **Latin Revolution Dance Academy,** Mississauga. David Palombi, instructor
- **Let's Dance London,** London. Julia Cassis, instructor
- **Let Us Dance,** Toronto. Sergei Filushkin, instructor
- **London Salsa Academy,** London. Ross Todorovic, Milena Todorovic, instructors
- **London Salsa Dance Company,** London.

- **Mambo Fever Dance Alliance,** Toronto. Leah Duque, choreographer
- **Mandy's Dance,** Mississauga. Mandy Epprecht, principal & instructor
- **Midday Fix,** Toronto
- **Nuvitzo Dance Academy,** Hamilton. Sean Quinlan (artistic director) Ashley Brown, Dan Dubeckyj, Sanya Khan, German Simmon
- **Olé to Dance,** Oakville. Dania
- **Olympic Stars Dance Academy,** Vaughan. Aruna Bizokas, owner/instructor
- **O.N.E. Dance Centre,** London. Mike, instructor
- **Oscar Naranjo Productions,** Toronto and Markham. Oscar Naranjo, principal
- **Ottawa Latin Corner Dance Studio,** Ottawa
- **Ottawa Latin Souls,** Ottawa. Jeff, instructor
- **Queen's University Salsa Club,** Kingston.
- **Rhythm & Motion Dance Studio,** Toronto. Elizabeth Sadlowska, director. Sergei Filushkin, Tarek Marroushi, Linda Smith, instructors
- **Salchata Dance Academy,** Toronto. Sam Mardini, co-founder, co-director
- **Salsa & Sabor Colombian Dance Academy,** Toronto. Camila Cepeda, director/instructor; Kenny Rojas. instructor
- **Salsa Beats,** Barrie. Natasha & Freddy, instructors
- **Salsa Café,** Brampton. Gonzalo Olea, founder/manager/instructor
- **Salsa Dance Productions,** Toronto. Jill Hollingsworth, instructor
- **SalsaFanatics Dance School,** Ottawa
- **Salsa Fever Dance Studio,** Ottawa. Oscar, instructor
- **Salsaholics Anonymous,** Toronto. Sanam Devine, owner
- **Salsa to the Heart,** Toronto. Miguel Gutierrez, founder/instructor
- **Slyde Ballroom and DanceSport,** London, Sarnia. Jamie Lyndon, owner/founder
- **Smooth Latin Grooves Dance Studio,** Barrie. Norbert Wunn, owner/instructor
- **Soul2Sole Latin Dance Company,** Toronto, Vaughan
- **Star Dance Centre,** Toronto. Fiona Su, instructor
- **Step in Two Dance,** Ajax. Vladimir Suanez, owner/instructor

- **Steps Dance Studio,** Toronto. Jennifer Aucoin, Angelo De Torres, directors; Kathy De Torres, instructor
- **Tania Dance Connexion,** Toronto. Tania Wong, director
- **The Baila Boogaloo Dance Co.,** Toronto. Joaquin E. Martinez, artistic director/head choreographer; Darlene Wang, co-founder/principal
- **The Love of Salsa,** Ajax
- **The Salsa Dance Floor,** Mississauga. Rocco Michael, instructor
- **Toronto Dance**! Jim Groneau, owner/instructor
- **Toronto Dance Fridays,** Toronto
- **Toronto Dance Inc.,** Toronto. Chuan Chee, president/instructor. Melvin Baird, Darren Baird, Lisa Fender, Bill Forsythe, Iryna Iaremchuk, Gorete Almeida
- **Toronto Dance Salsa,** Toronto. Aleksander Saiyan, principal
- **United Salseros,** Toronto. Teddy, Jesse, Jody, Kevin, instructors
- **York Dance Academy,** Aurora, Newmarket, Stouffville. Angela Tucker, artistic director/owner, Joel Wood, Juan Alberto, instructors

## Prince Edward Island

- **DownStreet Dance Studio,** Charlottetown.

## Québec

- **Arthur Murray Dance Centers,** Dollard-des-Ormeaux, Laval, Montréal, Québec City
- **Baila Productions,** Laval, West Island, L'Île-Perrot.
- **Como Mango Dance Studio,** Montréal
- **Concordia University Recreation,** Montréal
- **Confidanse Inc.,** Montréal.
- **Corinne & Victor,** Montréal. Corinne Tardieu, Victor Alexis, instructors
- **Dance Conmigo,** Montréal. Alain Guillot, Cheryl Williams, instructors
- **École de Danse Grenier,** Varennes. Andrée Grenier, Manon Grenier, co-owners/instructors
- **École Quartier Latin Montreal Dansesport School,** Montréal. Alina, Maxim, instructors
- **Espaces Des Arts,** Montréal

- **Hot Latin Salsa Dance Courses,** Montréal
- **Julie Bergeron Danse Sociale,** Vimont (Laval). Julie Bergeron, principal
- **Hot Latin Salsa Dance Studio,** Verdun
- **Latin Groove Dance & Fitness,** Montréal. Sandra Campanelli, owner
- **L'École de Danse de Québec,** Québec
- **Le Social Salsa Dance Studio,** Montréal.
- **Salsa Antonio Salatti Dance Schools,** Montréal
- **Salsa Brossard Rive-Sud,** Brossard
- **Salsa Etc.,** Montréal. Alberto Azpuro, instructor
- **San Tropez Dance Centre,** Montréal. Sonia Kyriacou, co-founder/artistic director, Moris Alvarenga, co-founder/master instructor
- **Strazzero Latin Dance Academy/Studio 2720 Canada,** Montréal. Mathieu Casavant, director
- **Studio Blue Mambo Dance Studio,** Sainte-Foy
- **Studio Musique et Danse,** Verdun
- **Studio Salsa Attitude,** Québec City

## Saskatchewan

- **BKS YXE,** Saskatoon. Leah Frei, Leo Liendo, principals/instructors
- **Dance Class Saskatoon,** Saskatoon.
- **Danza Morena Latin Dance Academy,** Saskatoon. Carmen Gonza, principal. Maria Balmeo, Sacha Favel, Solange Rego, Deldra Toner, instructors
- **Regina Salseros**, Regina. Will Siguenza, founder/instructor. Jennifer Giatras, Flany B., instructors
- **Saskatoon Salsa Dance Co.,** Saskatoon. Kimberley Parent, principal. Robynn Dupuis, Kristina Bykowy, Ervin Kormos, Mariana Lessa, Ludovic Piejos, instructors

# Square Dancing

## Alberta

- **Acey Pluses**, Calgary

- **Athabasca River Dancers,** Athabasca
- **Banff Trailers,** Calgary
- **Boyle Twilight Twirlers,** Boyle
- **Brownfield Prairie Sunset Dancers,** Brownfield
- **Camrose Rose City Swingers,** Camrose
- **Caribooters,** Lac La Hache
- **Central Squares Plus,** Red Deer
- **Country Cousins,** Sherwood Park
- **Country Shiners,** Edmonton
- **Crazee 8's Squares,** Lethbridge
- **Crossfire Plus,** Edmonton
- **Dots & Dashers,** Calgary
- **Double As – A2 Club,** Calgary
- **Double Diamond Dancers,** Edmonton
- **Edmonton Singles Squares,** Edmonton
- **Evansburg Square Dancers,** Evansburg
- **Friday Plus,** Calgary
- **Golden Circle Square Dancers,** Red Deer
- **Happy Homesteaders,** Leduc
- **Hi-Land Swingers,** Calgary
- **Hinton Square Dance Club,** Hinton
- **Kick-a-Poo-Kids,** Bon Accord
- **Lethbridge Tape Squares Club,** Lethbridge
- **Lloydminster Chain 'N' Circle Club,** Esther Boyce 780-872-2493
- **Luke's & Lucys,** Edmonton
- **Olds Calico Capers,** Olds
- **Parkland Belles & Beaux Squares,** Parkland
- **Plamondon Valley Dancers,** Plamondon
- **Prairie Wind Dancers,** Medicine Hat
- **Queens & Jacks,** Calgary
- **Rainbow Country Dancers,** Nanton
- **Red Deer Square Dance Club,** Red Deer

- **Rockyview Ramblers,** Airdrie
- **Rocky Whirlaways Square Dance Club,** Rocky Mountain House
- **Sandholm Crossroad Dancers,** Sandholm
- **Wandering Squares**, Various locations
- **West Edmonton Promenades,** Edmonton
- **Western Square Dance Club,** Calgary
- **Whitecourt Whirlers,** Whitecourt
- **Wheatland Whirlers,** Strathmore
- **Yellowhead Square Dance Club,** Edson

## British Columbia

- **Abbotsford Grand Squares,** Abbotsford
- **Abbotsford Swinging Hubs,**
- **Arthur Murray Dance Studio,** Vancouver
- **Brent's Bunch,** Burnaby
- **Chilliwack Rhythm Reelers,** Chilliwack
- **Chuckwagon 8s,** Burnaby
- **Circle & Squares,** Nanaimo
- **Circle Eights,** Quesnel
- **Country Cousins,** Victoria
- **Century House,** New Westminster
- **Delta Sundancers,** Surrey teens
- **Dance A Rounds,** Victoria
- **Don's Plus,** Salmon Arm
- **Drifting Squares,** Vanderhoof
- **Enderby River Dancers,** Enderby
- **4 Ways Family Dance Club,** Salmon Arm
- **Frontier Twirlers Square Dance Club,** Colwood
- **Gold Classic Dancers,** Kamloops
- **Guys 'N' Gals,** Aldergrove
- **Kamloops Square Dancers,** Kamloops

- **Mavericks,** Victoria
- **Mile Zero Grand Squares, Dawson Creek**
- **Motiv8ors,** Burnaby
- **Nelson's Tuesday Plus,** Vernon
- **Northern Twisters,** Prince George
- **Ocean Waves,** Courtenay-Comox
- **Promenaders Square Dance Club,** Victoria
- **Quick Steppers,**
- **Rainbow Rounders,** Victoria
- **Ripple Rockets,** Campbell River
- **Royal Swingers,** Burnaby
- **Rhythm Rounds,** Vernon
- **Salmon Arm Squares,** Salmon Arm
- **Salty Wheels,** Salt Spring Island
- **Skeena Squares,** Terrace
- **Squares Across the Border,**
- **Stampede Whirlaways,** Williams Lake
- **Star Country Squares,** Vernon
- **Star Dusters,** Powell River
- **Stardowners,** New Westminster
- **Star Twirlers Square Dance Club,** Victoria
- **Swinging Hubs,** Aldergrove
- **Swinging Singles Square Dance Club,** Burnaby
- **Surrey Square Wheelers,** Langley
- **Thompson Valley Stars,** Kamloops
- **Travelling Squares,** Nanaimo
- **The Mavericks Square Dance Club, Victoria**
- **Town & Country Dancers,** Maple Ridge
- **Track IIs,** Courtenay-Comox
- **TW Twirlers Square Dance Club,** Delta
- **Valley Promenaders,**
- **Wesburn Wranglers,** Burnaby

- **Westsyde Squares**, West Kelowna
- **Westsyde Youth Team Dance Club,** Kelowna
- **Wheel Arounds,** Lady Smith
- **Wheel Arounds,** Nanaimo
- **Wheeling 8s,** Surrey
- **White Rockers,** White Rock

## Manitoba

- **B&B Rounds,** Winnipeg
- **Beausejour Swinging Squares,**
- **Brandon Circle Eights,**
- **Crazy 8s,**
- **Diamond Squares,**
- **Grand Squares,**
- **Hamiota Happy Hustlers**
- **Paws & Taws**
- **Portage Pairs & Squares,**
- **St. Vital Swingers,**
- **Swan Valley Hoedowners,** Swan River
- **TJ's Square Dance Club,** Winnipeg
- **The Pas Square Dancers,**
- **Whirlaway Westerners,** Winnipeg
- **Xtenders,** Brandon

## New Brunswick

- **Beaus & Belles,** Quispamsis
- **Browns Flats Beaus & Belles,**
- **Country Cousins,** Burnt Church
- **East Coast As,** Quispamsis
- **Elm Tree Square & Round Dance Club,** Fredericton

- **Fundy Wheelers,** Grand Bay-Westfield
- **Hampton Hoedowners,** Sussex
- **Hoban's Heroes,** Riverview
- **Oromocto Pioneers,** Oromocto
- **Starlight Promenaders,** Clifton Royal
- **Sussex Corner Dance Club,** Sussex Corner
- **Tantramar Twirlers,** Sackville
- **Town & Country Squares,** St. Stephen
- **Washademoak Swingers,** Shannon
- **Woodstock Wheelers,** Northhampton

# Newfoundland & Labrador

No square-dancing clubs identified.

## Nova Scotia

- **Apple Valley Dancers,** Lawrencetown
- **Coordinators Plus,** Dartmouth
- **Cumberland Twirlers,** Nappan
- **Fun Time Rounds,** Lake Echo
- **Fundy Squares,** Wilmot
- **Harmony Squares,** Dartmouth
- **Highland Squares,** Westville
- **Lake City Swingers,** Dartmouth
- **Mapleleaf Whirlaways,** (in) Cape Breton Region
- **Motivators,** Lawrencetown
- **Parkland at the Lakes Seniors,** Dartmouth
- **Sail Sets,** Rockingham
- **South Shore Squares,** Bridgewater
- **Star Dusters (Benny Slade's Starduster Square Dance Club)** Dartmouth

- **Young Country Dancers,** Melvern Square

## Ontario

- **A2 Teach,** Burlington
- **Afternoon Rounds,** St. Catharines
- **Amethyst Square Dance Club,** Thunder Bay
- **Arrowhead Squares,** Etobicoke (Toronto)
- **Blue Mountain Promenaders,** Collingwood
- **Bay Waves,** Constance Bay
- **Centennial Beavers,** London
- **Chain Reactors,** Guelph
- **Charmin' Promenaders,** Cornwall
- **Country Squares,** Lucknow
- **Clinton - Huron Happy Hearts,** Clinton
- **Crazy A's,** Ottawa
- **Daytime A1 Teach,** Cambridge
- **Daytime Advanced,** Brampton.
- **Denim N Lace,** Flesherton
- **Fort Frances Pairs and Squares,** Fort Frances
- **Gateway Gliders,** North Bay
- **Glengarry Tartans,** Alexandria
- **Grand Squares,** Elora
- **Grenville Gremlins,** Kemptville
- **Guys N Dolls,** Kitchener
- **Hanover - Happy twirlers**
- **Happy Hoppers,** Newmarket
- **Harbour Lites,** Prescott
- **Horseman Squares C112,** Waterloo
- **Huron Bruce Swingers,** Lucknow
- **Jubilee Rounds,** St. Jacobs
- **Kanata Squares,** Kanata

- **Kawartha Clover Leafs,** Lindsay
- **Lakeshore Waves,** Port Hope.
- **Lift Lock Squares,** Peterborough.
- **Limestone Dancers,** Kingston
- **Lockits,** Black's Corners.
- **M&B Rounds,** Thunder Bay
- **Kawartha Clover Leafs,** Lindsay
- **Meri Squares,** Ottawa
- **Minesing Midhurst Squares**
- **Mississippi Squares,** Carleton Place
- **Mississauga Sunday Brunch**
- **Napanee Pioneers,** Napanee
- **Opeongo Squares,** Barrys Bay
- **Oshawa Squares,** Oshawa
- **Otonabee Squares,** Peterborough
- **Ottawa Date Squares,** Ottawa
- **Pioneers Square Dance Club,** Napanee
- **Promenaders Square Dance Club,** Thunder Bay
- **Quinte Twirlers,** Belleville
- **Rainbow Squares,** Niagara Falls
- **Rhythm Rounds,** London
- **Riverside Gypsy Squares,** Brockville
- **Royal City Squares,** Guelph
- **Silver Streak,** Woodstock
- **Sound Steppers,** Owen Sound.
- **Star Promenaders,** Marlbank
- **Sunshine Squares,** Ottawa
- **Swinging Bs,** Cornwall
- **Swinging Duos,** Strathroy.
- **Thames Valley Dance Club,** Woodstock
- **Triangle Squares,** Toronto
- **The Bay Waves,** Constance Bay

- **The Sunday Brunch,** Mississauga
- **Village Squares,** Orleans
- **Waterdown Village Squares,** Waterdown
- **West St. Catharines Older Adult Centre,** St Catharines
- **Wheel N Dealers Square Dance,** Clinton.

## Prince Edward Island

No square dance clubs identified.

## Quebéc

- **Circles and Squares,** Pointe Claire
- **Maple Country Swingers,** Asbestos
- **Montréal Acey Deuceys,** Pointe Claire
- **Seaway Swingers,** Greenfield Park
- **Swinging Stars,** Dollard-des-Ormeaux

## Saskatchewan

- **Battle River Cloggers,** North Battleford
- **Cotton Capers Square Dance Club,** Saskatoon
- **Estevan Diamond Dancers & Hitch & Hike Twirlers,** Estevan
- **DanceLand,** Manitou Beach
- **Fiske Funtastics,** Fiske
- **Happy Hearts Square & Round Dance Club,** Regina
- **Karousels Round Dance Club,** Saskatoon
- **Kindersley Whirls & Twirls,** Kindersley
- **Lloydminster Chain 'n' Circle,** Lloydminster
- **Park Swingers Square & Round Dance Club,** Yorkton
- **Renz Rounds,** Swift Current
- **Rhythm E's Round Dance Club**
- **River City Squares,** Saskatoon
- **Swift Current Square Dance Club,** Swift Current
- **Town 'N' Country Squares,** Moose Jaw

- **Unity Wagon Wheels**, Unity
- **Whitmore Pioneers Square Dance Club**, Regina

# Round Dancing

## Alberta

- **Circle Chase Rounds**, Innisfail
- **Cue Steps**, Calgary
- **Fun Steps**, Edmonton
- **Kensington Strollers**, Edmonton
- **Lacombe Round Dance Club**, Lacombe
- **Merry Go Round Dance Club**, Calgary
- **Rocky Mountain House Whirlaway Rounds**, Rocky Mountain House
- **Wild Rose Country Dancers**, Edmonton

## British Columbia

- **Amalgam-Eighters**, Lantzville
- **Guys 'N' Gals**, Aldergrove
- **Dance A Rounds**, Victoria
- **Island Gems Round Dance Club**, Lantzville
- **Island Gems Round Dance Club**, Nanaimo
- **R&R Rounders**, Penticton
- **Rhythm Bs**, Surrey
- **Sand Dollars**, Parksville
- **Swinging Singles Square Dance Club**, Burnaby
- **Wesburn Wranglers**, Burnaby
- **Wheel Arounds**, Lady Smith
- **Wheel Arounds**, Nanaimo

## Ontario

- **Capital Carousels**, Ottawa
- **Limestone Dancers**, Kingston

- **Stepping Out Rounds**, Ottawa

## Manitoba

- **B & B Rounds**, Winnipeg

## New Brunswick

- **Beaus & Belles**, Saint John
- **Capital City Ballroom Sequence & Round Dance Club**, Fredericton
- **Elm Tree Squares**, Fredericton
- **Sussex Corner Dance Club**, Sussex Corner
- **Town & Country Squares**, St. Stephen

## Newfoundland & Labrador

No round dancing clubs identified.

## Nova Scotia

- **Fun Time Rounds**, Dartmouth

## Prince Edward Island

No round dancing clubs identified.

## Québec

No round dancing clubs identified.

## Saskatchewan

- **Fiske Funtastics**, Fiske
- **Karousels Round Dance Club**, Saskatoon
- **ParkSwingers Square & Round Dance Club**, Yorkton
- **Hub City Square and Round Dance Assn.**, Saskatoon
- **ParkSwingers Square & Round Dance Club**, Yorkton

- **Renz's Rounds,** Swift Current
- **Happy Hearts Square & Round Dance Club,** Regina
- **Rhythm E's Round Dance Club,** Regina
- **Whitmore Pioneers Square & Dance Club,** Grand Coulee
- **Sun City Square & Round Dance Club,** Townsville

# About the Author

John Yuen is an associate member of the Canadian Association of Journalists and the Investigative Reporters & Editors organization. He has freelanced for publications including *Communication World, Marketing,* and *Human Resources Professional.* He co-authored *Thinking Hands* (2015). As well, he sometimes dances from "dusk 'til dawn," and is an itinerant social ballroom and Latin dance instructor. A CAM (Communication Advertising Marketing Foundation) diploma holder in public relations from the U.K., he obtained undergraduate and graduate degrees from the Universities of Ryerson, York and Carleton. He also won a Silver Award from the Information Officers' Forum in Toronto for communications strategy and marketing.

# References

## Telephone Interviews

- Argentini, Giorgio. Telephone interview. 13 August 2020
- Asgary, Minoo & Omar Kazi.. Telephone interview. 8 October 2020
- Borshch, Anna. Telephone interview. 28 August 2020
- Borstein, Hindy. Telephone interview. 8 October 2020
- Brailean, Vivian. Telephone interview. 1 February 2021
- Brossard, Liboire ("Lee"). Telephone interview. 23 February 2021
- Campbell, Dorothy. Telephone interview. 1 February 2021
- Carleton, Alexander, Telephone interview, 8 December 2020
- Chandarana, Nina. Telephone interview. 20 February 2021
- Cheng, Fred. Telephone interview. 23 August 2020
- Cheung, Ying. Telephone interview. 13 September 2020
- Chirca, Cristina. Telephone interview. 24 February 2021
- Chow, Juliana. Telephone interview. 1 September 2020
- Clark, Larry & Marg. Telephone interview. 24 February 2021
- Dina, Cristina Amalia, Telephone interview. 13 November 2020
- Dubé, Michel, Telephone interview. 13 August 2020
- Dyke, Eleanor & Dean Little. Telephone interview. 9 October 2020
- Epprecht, Mandy. Telephone interview. 16 August 2020
- Evans, Karen & Jim. Telephone interview. 9 October 2020
- Franks, David & Diane Ternan. Telephone interview. 18 November 2020

- Evelyn, Gregory. Telephone interview, 23 August 2020
- Fulton, Mary. Telephone interview. 12 August 2020
- Greenhill, Judy. Telephone interview. 17 September 2020
- Hill, Colin & Valery. Telephone interview. March 2 2021
- Holliday-Tucker, Sandra. Telephone interview. 26 October 2020
- Kanyo, Ginette & John. Telephone interview. 4 October 2020
- Keating, Nella & Patrick. Telephone interview. 20 October 2020
- Lajoie, Bert & Shirley. Telephone interview. 8 October 2020
- Leong, Ivan & Santha. Telephone Interview. 19 November 2020
- Loomis, John. Telephone interview. 25 February 2021
- Lubberts, Dale & J. Jelies. Telephone interview. 30 October 2020
- Mastrandrea, Pat. Telephone interview. 20 October 2020
- McCormack, Eric. Telephone interview. 25 August 2020
- Meinecke, Alice. Telephone interview. 16 September 2020
- Meyer, Merv. Telephone interview. 11 February 2021
- Morina, Vahide. Telephone interview. 8 March 2021
- Nelson, Steve. Telephone interview. 23 August 2020
- Panacci, Dominic. Telephone interview. 21 August 2020
- Parks, Paul & Theresa. Telephone interview. 27 February 2021
- Price, Ralph. Telephone interview. 12 September 2020
- Russell, Bill. Telephone interview. 8 September 2020
- Saiyan, Aleksander. Telephone interview. 1 September 2020
- Sato, Leo. Telephone interview. 20 August 2020
- Sedman, Bud. Telephone interview. 6 January 2021
- Silverman, Arkady. Telephone interview, 30 August 2020
- Solomon, Corey. Telephone interview. 18 August 2020
- Sommer, Martina. Telephone interview. 15 February 2021
- Stanfield, Barry & Esther. Telephone interview 14 October 2020
- Stanfield, Esther. Telephone interview 14 October 2020
- Stone, Kathryn. Telephone interview. 27 February 2021
- Stradling, Cindy. Telephone Interview. 18 November 2020
- Szymczak, Monika. Telephone interview. 20 August 2020
- Tan, Timothy. Telephone interview. 17 September 2020
- Tucker, Silas, Telephone Interview. 26 October 2020
- Vanderaa, Vaunda. Telephone interview. 1 February 2021
- W., Andria, Telephone interview. 28 November 2020

- White, Marjorie. Telephone Interview. 26 August 2020
- Willems, Jacinta (Dr.) Telephone interview. 24 February 2021

Numerous other persons within and outside the social dance community participated informally by being interviewed throughout the research period of this project. The author conducted the interviews.

# Correspondence from Individuals

Dobrynina, Maria. Email to the author. 28 August 2020
Forbes-Anderson, Faye. Email to the author. 16 July 2020
Jestin, Jerry. Email to the author. 6 January 2021
Lam, Patricia. Email to the author. 8 March 2021
McKay, Louise. Email to the author. 8 September 2020
Nakamura, Maryrose. Email to the author. 28 August 2020
Okazawa, Tadahiro. Email to the author. 8 September 2020

# Correspondence from Organizations

**Belleville**, City of, Ontario. Email from Tanya Grierson. 22 July 2020
**Bradford West Gwillimbury,** Town of, Ontario. Email from Nancy Shortill-Thatcher. 5 February 2021
**Caledon**, Town of, Ontario. Email from Parm Chohan. 12 August 2020
**Cambridge**, City of, Ontario. Email from Colleen Lichti. 10 July 2020
**Edmonton**, City of, Alberta. Email from Alex Hamilton. 14 July 2020
**East Gwillimbury**, Town of, Ontario. Email from Laura Hanna, 14 July 2020
**Halifax**, City of, Nova Scotia. Email from Maggie-Jane Spray. 13 July 2020
**King,** Township of, Ontario. Email from Adam Viola. 22 July 2020
**Kitchener**, City of, Ontario. Email from LoriAnn Palubeski. 14 July 2020
**Lake Country**, District of, British Columbia. Email from Karen Miller. 15 July 2020
**Maple Ridge**, City of, British Columbia. Email from Naomi Evans. 21 July 2020
**Newmarket,** Town of, Ontario. Email from Janis Luttrell, 2 June 2021
**North Vancouver**, City of, British Columbia. Email from Jeremy Neill. 19 August 2020
**Pointe-Claire,** City of, Québec. Email from Marie-Pier Paquette-Séguin. 6 August 2020
**Red Deer County**, Municipal District of, Alberta. Email from Jerry Jestin.

6 January 2021.
**Salmon Arm**, City of, British Columbia. Email from Donna Flatman and Darby Boyd, 13 & 17 July 2020
**Toronto,** City of, Toronto. Email from Andrea Gonsalves, 25 February 2021
**Val-des-Monts**, Québec. Email from Patricia Fillet. 22 July 2020
**Ville de Pointe-Claire**, Québec. Email from Marie-Pier Paquette-Séguin, 6 August 2020
**Westmount**, City of, Québec. Email from Claude Danis. 28 August 2020
**Whitchurch-Stouffville**, Town of, Ontario. Email from Barb Armstrong, 5 July 2020
**Windsor, City of**, Ontario. Email from Scott Bisson, Joey Ouellette and Cathy Masterson. 20 July 2020

# Bibliography

Anon. "Arts and dance related evaluations: Dancing with Parkinson's," https://torontoevaluation.ca/centre/?page_id=74

Anon. "Atlantic Canada," The Canada Guide. https://thecanadaguide.com/places/atlantic-canada/

Anon. https://www.canadahistory.ca/explore/arts-culture-society/toot-sweet-when-jazz-ruled-Montréal.

Anon. https://www.canadiandancesportfederation.ca

Anon. "Ball Dress," Encyclopedia of Clothing and Fashion , Vol.1. New York: Charles Scribner's Sons, 2005.

Anon. "Canada's entertainment in the 1920s,"https://prezi.com/hb5dzkksh_zgp/canadas-entertainment-in-the-1920s/#:~:text=Dances%20such%20as%20the%20charleston.%2C%%20and%20Lindy%20Hop.

Anon. "Drum Dance." http://native-drums.ca/en/music/drum-dance/, accessed 1 July 2020.

Anon. Duke Ellington & His Orchestra Concert Setlist at Trianon Ballroom, Regina on June 29, 1954. | setlist.fm.

Anon. https://www.gluckstein.com/introducing-wheel-dance-wheelchair-dancesport/

Anon. "Great Depression in Canada." https://en.wikipedia.org/wiki/Great_Depression_in_Canada.

Anon. "History of radio broadcasting. In Canada." History of broadcasting in Canada - Wikipedia

Anon. "Introducing wheel dance & wheelchair dancesport" https://www.gluckstein.com/introducing-wheel-dance-wheelchair-dancesport/

Anon. "Jane Austen's world," https://janeaustensworld.wordpress.com/2011/09/30/an-18th-century-ladys-toilette-hours-of-leisurely-dressing-and-private-affairs/

Anon. "Mart Kenney and His Western Gentlemen." Mart Kenney and His Western Gentlemen | The Canadian Encyclopedia

Anon. "Montréal in roaring twenties," https://www.canadahistory.ca/explore/arts-culture-society/toot-sweet-when-jazz-ruled-Montréal

Anon. "New styles influenced by dances." The Toronto World, 13 January 1914, vol. XXXIV, no. 12.

Anon. "Open morris: A short history of morris dancing," https://open-morris.org/morris-dancing/

Anon. http://squaredancemb.com/

Anon. "Sunny Fry Orchestra engaged for board of trade dance," Bassano Recorder, 4 April 1940.

Anon. "Wheelchair Dance Classes" http://chancedancecentre.com/

Alberta Teachers' Association (The). "Native Dance." http://native-dance.ca/en/culture/mikmaq/who-we-are/

_____. "First Nations, Metis and Inuit Music and Dance," Stepping Stones. no.10.

Albertson, Karen. "Testimonials - What Educators, Parents and Students are Saying!" Welcome to Join the Dance (Canada)

Anastakis, Dimitry. "Industrialization in Canada," The Canadian Encyclopedia, https://www.thecanadianencyclopedia.ca/en/article/industrialization

Bailar Productions. https://www.bailarproductions.com/dance

Bailey, Nathan. An Universal Etymological English Dictionary, 1742.

Ballroom Dance Studios. http://ballroomdancestudios.ca

Barrick, Simon, Lindsay Kavanaugh, Keith Macfarlane and Theodore Christou. The history of dance education in 20th century Ontario schools: 1950 to 2010. 19 November 2012,

https://www.curriculumhistory.org/Studies_in_Curriculum_History_and_Educational_Philosophy/Select_Subjects_in_the_History_of_Ontario_Education_files/The%20History%20of%20Dance%20Education%20in%2020th%20Century%20Ontario%20Schools.pdf, accessed 25 November 2020.

Biehn, Janice. "Let's dance," Chatelaine (English ed.), December 1995.

Bonvillain, Nancy. "The Mi"kmaqs," Native Nations: Cultures and Histories of Native North America. New York: Rowman & Littlefield, 2016.

Brittanica, "Royal Control." https://www.britannica.com/place/Canada/Royal-control

_____ . "Bourree." https://www.britannica.com/art/country-dance

_____ . "Country dance: British dance." https://www.britannica.com/art/country-dance

_____ . "Passepied dance." https://www.britannica.com/art/passepied

_____ . "Rigaudon dance." https://www.britannica.com/art/rigaudon

_____ . "Royal control." https://www.britannica.com/place/Canada/Royal-control

Buckland, Theresa Jill. "From the artificial to the natural body: social dancing in Britain, 1900-1914," Eds. https://link.springer.com/chapter/10.1057/9780230354487_5

Alexandra Carter & Rachel Fensham. Dancing naturally: nature, neo-classicism and modernity in early twentieth-century dance. London: Palgrave Macmillan, 2011.

Canadian Encyclopedia (The). "Economic History of Western Canada," https://www.thecanadianencyclopedia.ca/en/article/economic-history-of-western-Canada

CBC (Canadian Broadcasting Corporation). "Demonstrators rally, march, dance in Toronto to show support for Wet'suwet'en hereditary chiefs," https://www.cbc.ca/news/canada/toronto/rally-march-dance-wetsuweten-hereditary-chiefs-toronto-support-1.5472838, accessed 3 December 2020

CBC News. "Neurological patients learn to tango in Halifax: Social sharing: Dancers hve Alzheimer's and Parkinson's disease". https://www.cbc.ca/news/canada/nova-scotia/neurological-patients-learn-to-tango-in-halifax-1.2433114

Calgary Dance Club (The). Email. 28 November 2020.

Campbell, Patricia. "18th century or colonial dances." https://countrydancecaller.com/18th-century-or-colonial-dances/

Canada Council for the Arts. Summary of The Canada Dance Mapping Study, | 1 December 2016.

_____. Findings from Yes, I dance: A survey of who dances in Canada. Ottawa: 21 July 2014. https://canadacouncil.ca/research/research-library/2014/07/findings-from-yes-i-dance-a-survey-of-who-dances-in-canada

_____ & Ontario Arts Council. Findings from Yes I Dance: A survey of who dances in Canada: Final Report. Executive_Summary_Yes_I_Dance_EN.pdf, accessed 8 September 2020.

Canadian DanceSport Federation. https://www.canadiandancesportfederation.ca

Canadian Press (The). "U.S. society recommends British style of dancing," The Globe and Mail, 6 August 1957.

_____. "Bad for discipline: women teachers must not teach boy students dancing," The Globe, 13 December 1935.

Carroll, Lewis and John Tenniel. Alice's Adventures in Wonderland, London: SDE Classics, 2019.

Champlain Society for the Government of Ontario (The). The town of York 1815-1834: A further collection of documents of early Toronto. University of Toronto Press, 1966.

Confederacy of Mainland Mi'kmaq (The). Kekina'muek (Learning), October 2007. https://native-land.ca/wp/wp-content/uploads/2018/06/Mikmaq_Kekinamuek-Manual.pdf

Conniff, Richard. Strange Behaviors: Cool Things from the Natural and Human Worlds. https://strangebehaviors.wordpress.com/2018/11/06/20000-year-old-cave-art-from-borneo-depicts-humans-dancing/, accessed 4 December 2020.

Cook, Ramsay. The Voyages of Jacques Cartier. Toronto: University of Toronto Press.

Cooke, Maud C. "Social etiquette, or manners and customs of polite society: Containing rules of etiquette for all occasions …," London, ON: McDermid & Logan, 1896.

Cooper, Cynthia. Magnificent entertainments: fancy dress balls of Canada's Governors General 1876-1898. Fredericton: Goose Lane Editions; Hull, PQ: Canada Museum of Civilization, 1997.

Craig, Gerald M. Upper Canada: The formative years 1784-1841. Toronto: McClelland and Stewart. 1963.

Cresswell, Tim. 'You cannot shake that shimmie here': Producing mobility on the dance floor. Cultural Geographies, 13(1), pp.55– 77. 2006. https://doi.org/10.1191/1474474006eu350oa, accessed 7 December 2020.

Crisp, Freda. Dance in polite society Hamilton, Canada West, 1840-1860. MFA thesis. Toronto: York University, 1991. https://elibrary.ru/item.asp?id=5824816

Crossley, H.T. A practical discussion of the parlor dance, the theatre, the cards. Toronto: William Briggs, 1895, p.15.

Cuesteps Round Dance Club. Calgary. https://rounddancecalgary.com/about-us/, accessed 6 September 2020.

Dahm, Dorothy. "The Beginnings of Square Dancing in North America." https://swosda.ca/history

Daugherty, Fred. "The 'animal dancers' so wild they were banned from the White House: when a 'turkey trot' craze swept the nation in the 1910s, authority figures panicked". https://www.history.com/news/banned-animal-dance-turkey-trot-woodrow-wilson, accessed 29 September 2020

Dictionary of Canadian Biography. http://www.biographi.ca/en/bio/rocbert_de_la_morandiere_marie_elisabeth_3E.html

Doolittle, Lisa. "The Trianon and on: Reading mass social dancing in the 1930s and 1940s in Alberta, Canada." Dance Research Journal, Winter 2001, vol.33, no.2.

Drummond, Ian M. & Ford Macintosh, "Economic history of Central Canada," The Canadian Encyclopedia. https://www.thecanadianencyclopedia.ca/en/article/economic-history-of-central-canada

_____ . "Economic History of Western Canada," The Canadian Encyclopedia, https://www.thecanadianencyclopedia.ca/en/article/economic-history-of-western-Canada

E & R Ballroom Dance Studio. Newsletter for Sunday November 22,, 2020.

EKOS Research Associates Inc. Summary: findings from Yes I Dance: A survey of who dances in Canada: bringing the arts to life. Canada Council for the Arts, 21 July 2014, Executive_Summary_Yes_I_Dance_EN.pdf, accessed 8 September 2020.

_____. Final report: Findings from Yes I dance: A survey of who dances in Canada. Ottawa: Canada Council for the Arts, 21 July 2014, p.26.

Encyclopaedia of Clothing and Fashion, vol.1. New York: Charles Scribner's Sons, 2005.

Father La Jeune, report, The Jesuit Relations, 14 August 1636.

Firth, Edith G. "The Town of York `1815-1834," The Champlain Society for the Government of Ontario. The town of York 1815-1834: A further collection of documents of early Toronto. University of Toronto Press, 1966, front cover flap.

FitzHenry, Brianna. "1920s Canada." https://1920sentertainmentbybrianna.weebly.com/jazz-and-other-music.html

Franks, A.H. Social Dance: A Short History. London: Routledge and Keagan Paul, 1963.

Gadacz, René R. "Potlatch," The Canadian Encyclopedia, ,https://www.thecanadianencyclopedia.ca/en/article/potlatch

Gidney, Catherine. "The Dredger's daughter: courtship and marriage in the Baptist community of Welland, Ontario, 1934-1944." Labour (Committee on Canadian Labour History), pp.121-149.

Giménez-Llort, L. & Castillo-Mariqueo, L. " PasoDoble, a proposed dance/music for people with Parkinson's disease and their caregivers," Frontiers in Neurology, 12 November 2020. https://www.frontiersin.org/articles/10.3389/fneur.2020.567891/full

Giordano, Ralph G. Satan in the Dance Hall: Rev. John Roach Straton, Social Dancing, and Morality in 1920s New York City. Lanham, MD: The Scarecrow Press, Inc., 2008.

Godel, Sarah. "Ballroom: the dance that globalization built." Ballroom: The Dance That Globalization Built « Interrogating Dance Globalization (smith.edu).

Government of Nova Scotia. https://www.novascotia.com/see-do/attractions/port-royal-national-historic-site/1462, accessed 4 September 2020.

Gowder, Paul. "Pow Wow Calendar—experience native American culture at an event near you.". https://www.powwows.com/2020-pow-wow-calendar-experience-native-american-culture-at-an-event-near-you/

Green, Pamela and Norman Moyah. "Join the circle—the history and lore of the round dance," Windspeaker Publication, vol. 16, no.2, 1998. https://ammsa.com/publications/windspeaker/join-circle-history-and-lore-round-dance-0

Guillet, Edwin C. Early life in Upper Canada. Toronto: The Ontario Publishing Co. Ltd., 1933.

Hallowell, Gerald. "Prohibition in Canada," The Canadian Encyclopedia. | The Canadian Encyclopedia

Harris, Carolyn. "Royal tours of Canada" The Canadian Encyclopedia, https://www.thecanadianencyclopedia.ca/en/article/royal-tours.

Herdman, Jessica. The Cape Breton fiddling narrative: innovation, preservation, dancing. M.A. thesis, University of British Columbia, August 2008.

Hill, Kelly. "Impacts of COVID-19 on Canadian artists and independent cultural workers: Interim report based on I Lost My Gig Canada survey data as of May 27 [2020]," Hill Strategies Research Inc., Hamilton, ON. https://hillstrategies.com/2020/06/23/impacts-of-covid-19-on-canadian-artists-and-independent-cultural-workers/

Hill Strategies Research Inc. https://hillstrategies.com/2015/05/27/findings-from-yes-i-dance-a-survey-of-who-dances-in-canada/

Hobbs, Rev. Richard. The evils of the modern pleasure dance: A sermon preached by the Rev. Richard Hobbs: Colborne Street Methodist Church, Brantford: Strathroy, Ont.?

Hoefnagels, Anne. "Cree Round Dances," Native Dance. http://native-dance.ca/en/renewal/cree-round-dances/

Hunter, J.J., "The pleasure dance in its relation to religion and morality," Toronto: Methodist Book and Pub. House, 1881. p.11.

Innis, Mary Quayle, ed. Mrs. Simcoe's diary. Toronto: Macmillan of Canada, 1965.

Inuvialuit Regional Corporation (The). https://www.irc.inuvialuit.com/about-irc

KV Ballroom Dancing (Studio) https://www.kvballroomdancing.com

Kalbach, Warren E., "Population of Canada," The Canadian Encyclopedia, https://www.thecanadianencyclopedia.ca/en/article/population

Kallmann, Helmut. Canadian Encyclopedia. English ed., Toronto: Historica Canada, 2019. https://seaerch.proquest.com/docview/2316376441/4AD-FBEFEF0D7475EPQ/3?accountid=31255

Knowles, Mark. The wicked waltz and other scandalous dances: Outrage at couple dancing in the 19th and early 20th centuries. Jefferson, NC: McFarland & Company, Inc. 2009.

Knowles, Patricia. "Dance education in American public schools," Bulletin of the Council for Research in Music Education, Summer, 1993, no.17.

Kracht, Benjamin R. "Kiowa Powwows: Tribal Identity Through the Continuity of the Gourd Dance," Great Plains Research, vol 4, no.2, August 1994.

Latindance.net. Montréal: https://www.latindance.net/language/en/health-safety/

Library and Archives Canada. Daily Life - Library and Archives Canada (bac-lac.gc.ca)

_____. "Daily Life in New France." http://www.canadahistoryproject.ca/1663/1663-14-daily-life.html

_____. "Survival," https://www.bac-lac.gc.ca/eng/discover/exploration-settlement/new-france-new-horizons/Pages/survival.aspx

Ling, Jan, R. Schenck and L. Shenck A History of European Folk Music, Rochester, N.Y.: University of Rochester Press, 1997.

Linteau, Paul-Andre, quoted in Iro Tembeck,. "Dancing in Montréal: seeds of a choreographic history," The Journal of the Society of Dance History Scholars, vol.5, no.2, Fall 1994.

Lockerby, Earle "Ancient Mi'kmaq customs: A Shaman's Revelations." Semantics Scholar, Stanford, ON. https://pdfs.semanticscholar.org/7335/0ed533ae3589b8e40a138a90c160b072d7c1.pdf

MUN Ballroom & Latin Dance Club. St. John's, Newfoundland & Labrador. https://www.facebook.com/groups/6027805871/

Mackie, John. "This week in history, 1938: Vancouver's first music star returns home to play the hotel Vancouver," Vancouver Sun, 21 October 2016. https://vancouversun.com/news/local-news/this-week-in-history-1938-vancouvers-first-music-star-returns-home-to-play-the-hotel-vancouver/

Magder Ted, Piers Handling, & Peter Morris, "Canadian Film History: 1896 to 1938,". The Canadian Encyclopedia https://www.thecanadianencyclopedia.ca/en/article/the-history-of-film-in-canada

Malleck, Dan. Try to control yourself: the regulation of public drinking in post-Prohibition Ontario 1927-44, Vancouver: University of British Columbia Press, 2013.

McDonald, Anne. Miss Confederation: The diary of Mercy Anne Coles. Toronto: Dundurn, 2017.

McGill Newsroom press release. "Shall we dance: Doing the tango improves the aging brain," Montreal: McGill University. 23 November 2005. https://www.mcgill.ca/newsroom/channels/news/shall-we-dance-1760

McMains, Juliet. Glamour Addiction: Inside the American ballroom dance industry, Middletown, CT: Wesleyan University Press, 2006.

McNamara, Helen. "Dance bands," https://www.thecanadianencyclopedia.ca/en/article/dance-bands-emc.

Miller, Gray. "History of social dance." Lovetoknow Corp. Burlingame, CA. https://dance.lovetoknow.com/History_of_Social_Dance

Milonga Querida Ottawa. https://www.facebook.com/MilongaQueridaOttawa/

O'D, P. "Taking the tang out of tango," Saturday Night, Dec. 13, 1913.

Outevsky, David. Soviet bodies in Canadian dancesport: Cultural identities, embodied politics, and performances of resistance in three Canadian ballroom dance studios. PhD. diss., Toronto: York University, 2018.

P. o'D. "Taking the tang out of tango," Saturday Night, Dec. 13, 1913.

Paper. Jordan D. Native North American religious traditions: dancing for life. Westport, CT: 2007

Powers, Richard. http://socialdance.stanford.edu/powers/DancesTaught.htm

_____. https://socialdance.stanford.edu/Syllabi/jazz_age.htm

_____. "Teen dances of the 1950s" Teen Dances" of the 1950s (stanford.edu)

Pozo, Cal. Let's dance: the complete book and DVD of ballroom dance instruction for weddings, parties, fitness and fun. Long Island City, N.Y.: Harleigh Press, 2007

Rousseau, Karine. "Balls (In the 19th and early 20th centuries)." Montréal: McCord Museum. http://collections.musee-mccord.qc.ca/scripts/explore.php?Lang=1&tablename=theme&tableid=11&elementid=83__true&contentlong

Prosper, Kerry, J. McMillan and A.A. Davis. "Returning to Netukulimk: Mi'kmaq cultural and spiritual connections with resource stewardship and self-governance," The International Indigenous Policy Journal, vol. 2, no. 4, 2011.

Public Health Agency of Canada (Neurological health charities Canada (NHCC). Mapping connections: An understanding of neurological conditions in Canada. Ottawa: 2014. (cited 2017 July 12) Report no.: HP35-45/2014E-PDF

Radford, Ian. Royal spectacle: the 1860 visit of the Prince of Wales to Canada and the United States. Toronto: University of Toronto Press, 2004.

Ramsay, Janis. "Dance studios holding rolling protest at Barrie City Hall," Barrie Advance, 28 February 2021.

Reynolds, John L. Ballroom Dancing: The Romance, Rhythm and Style. San Diego: Laurel Glen. 1998.

Robinson, Amanda. "Indigenous regalia in Canada," The Canadian Encyclopedia. https://www.thecanadianencyclopedia.ca/en/article/indigenous-regalia-in-canada

Rousseau, Karine. "Balls (In the 19th and early 20th centuries)." Montréal: McCord Museum. http://collections.musee-accord.qc.ca/scripts/explore.php?Lang=1&tablename=theme&tableid=11&elementid=83__true&contentlong

Rust, Frances, Dance in Society: An analysis of the relationship between the social dance and society in England from the Middle Ages to the Present Day. London: Routledge & Kegan Paul, 1969.

Sable, Trudy and Julia Sable. "Who we are," Native Dance. http://nativedance.ca/en/culturs/mikmaq/who-we-are/

Smith, Mary Larratt. Young Mr. Smith in Upper Canada. Toronto: University of Toronto Press, 1980.

Spence, Cathryn. "For the love of dance: Aurele Bellivea's life has been defined by the romance of dance," The (Moncton) Times-Transcript, 25 June 1999.

Square and Round Dancers of South Western Ontario. https://swosda.ca/

Srigley, Katrina. Breadwinning daughters: young working women in a depression-era city, 1929-1939, Toronto: University of Toronto Press, 2010.

Stevens, Lys. Dancing across the land: a report on the Canada Dance Mapping Inventory: bringing the arts to life (Canada Council for the Arts), 30 July 2013.

Tembeck, Iro "Dancing in Montreal: Seeds of a choreographic history," The Journal of the Society of Dance History Scholars, vol. 5, no. 2, Fall 1994.

30-Up Club. Listserve@30-up.com 21 October 2020

Thorburn, Chris, www.kelownaballroom.com/about.html

Tjaden, Ted. "Ragtime music in Canada": http://www.ragtimepiano.ca/rags/can2.htm.

Toronto Dance Salsa. https://torontodancesalsa.ca/free5095/

Toronto Evaluation Centre, University of Toronto. "Arts and dance related evaluations: Dancing with Parkinson's," https://torontoevaluation.ca/centre/?page_id=74

Tulk, Janice E. Our strength is ourselves: Identity, status, and cultural revitalization among the Mi'kmaq in Newfoundland. PhD diss., July 2008.

UBC Dance Club. http://ubcdanceclub.com/online-classes/

UNB Libraries. Journals: Centre for Digital Scholarship. https://journals.lib.unb.ca/

Waite, P.B. The life and times of Confederation 1864-1867: Politics, newspapers and the union of British North America, 3rd ed. Montréal: Robin Brass Studio, Inc., 2010.

Wallace, James. "Prince Albert was first British royal to visit Canada in 1860," Toronto Sun. 2 July 2017.

Walmsley, Kevin B. and Robert S. Kossuth. "Fighting it out in nineteenth-century Upper Canada/Canada West: Masculinities and physical challenges." Journal of Sport History, vol.27, no.3, 2000.

Warner, Mary Jane, Toronto Dance Teachers: 1925-1925, Arts Inter-Media Canada/Dance Collection Danse Press. Toronto, 1995.

Warwick, WM, Canadian ten cent ball-room companion and guide to dancing, comprising rules of etiquette, hints on private parties, toilettes for the ball-room, etc. Also a synopsis of round and square dances: diction of French terms, etc. Toronto: WM Warwick, 1871.

Wason, Janet. "The Victorian era ball," in Selma L. Odom & Mary J. Warner. Canadian dance: Visions and stories. Toronto: Dance Collection Danse, 2004

Weekes, Daniel J. Gateways to Empire Québec and New Amsterdam to 1664. Bethlehem, PA.: Lehigh University Press, 2019.

Whitworth, Thomas A. A History of Sequence Dancing and Script List. Derbyshire, U.K.: T.A. Whitworth,1995

Wikipedia. "Ballroom Dancing". https://en.wikipedia.org/wiki/Ballroom_dance.

_____. "History of radio broadcasting. in Canada." History of broadcasting in Canada - Wikipedia

Willis, Cheryl M. Tapping the Apollo: the African American female tap dance duo salt and pepper. Jefferson, N.C.: McFarland & Company, Inc., 2016.

Wong, Carissa. "The roaring twenties." https://medium.com/@wong_carissa/the-roaring-twenties-13d375bb4085

Wyman, Max; M. Crabb & S.M. Donaldson. "Dance in Canada", The Canadian Encyclopedia. https://www.thecanadianencyclopedia.ca/index.php/en/article/dance-history

Young, Peter. Let's dance: A celebration of Ontario's dance halls and summer dance pavilions. Toronto: Natural Heritage/Natural History Inc., 2002.

# Mass Media

*Barrie Advance*, 28 February 2021
*Bassano Recorder*, 4 April 1940
*British Colonist*, 21 October 1845
*Canadian Stamp News*, 1864
*Chatelaine*, December 1995
*CBC News*, 3 March 2020
*Global News*, 19 October 2020
*The Daily Mail*, 18 March 1914.
*The Lethbridge Telegram*, 14 January 1918.
*The Globe*, 20 November 1849; 9 December 1913; 13 December 1935
*The Globe and Mail*, 6 August 1957
*The Leader-Post*, 11 March 1977
*The Lethbridge Telegram*, 1 January 1918
*The Moncton Times*-Transcript, 25 June 1999
*The Toronto World*, 13 January 1914
*The Vancouver Sun*, 29 December 1934; 21 October 2016
*Toronto Life*, 31 December 2020
*Toronto Sun*, 2 July 2017
*Saturday Night*, 13 December 1913
*The Wetaskiwin Times*, 19 January 1922

# Social Media

@MacleodLisa

# Index

30-Up Club, 86, 90, 95, 117, 163, 164, 186, 222
Abraham, Ilsa, 77, 78, 184
Adams, Mary, 163
Afro-Caribbean dances, 66, 136
Alberta Square & Round Dance Federation, 152
Anglehart, Carla, 114, 126
Antonov, Konstantine, 163, 183
Argentine tango, 110, 114
    ballroom tango, 66
    Duchess of Connaught, 67
    in Québec, 177
    Tango Short Film & Documentary Festival, 150
    Tangomania, 67
Argentine Tango Lab, 149, 174
Argentini, Giorgio, 24, 209
Armenian dances, 136
Arthur Murray Dance Centers, 82, 173, 174, 176, 181, 187, 191, 194
Arthur Murray International Inc, 165
Arts Nova Scotia, 130
Arual, Ellen, 64
Asgary, Minoo, 111, 118, 167, 209
Asian-Canadians, 142
Atlantic Ballroom competion, 141
Aucoin, Jennifer, 144, 194

B.C. Square & Round Dance Federation, 109
bachata, 25, 87, 88, 98, 110, 111, 114, 120, 125, 144
Balboa (dance), 80, 164
balls
    1876-1898, 58, 217
    grand ball, Oct 14, 1864, 56
    grand ball, Sept 1, 1864, 57
    grand ball, Sept 6, 1864, 57
    inaugural 1667, 38
    Prince Charles, 56
    state, 38, 67
    Victorian Era Ball 1897, 58
Baycrest/NBS dance course, 133
BC Emergency Health Services, 98
Belashov, Egor, 151, 183, 192
Belgo Building (Montreal), 134
Belleville, City of, 157, 158, 160, 202, 211
Bishun, Frank, 144, 192
BKS YXE (dance club), 87, 195
Blackpool Junior Dance Festival, 123
Blok, Rebecca, 96
Borshch, Anna, 24, 141, 209
Borstein, Hindy, 112, 209
Bouma, Jitka, 182, 191
Bracebridge, 98, 124

Bradford–West Gwillimbury, Town of, 103, 109
Brailean, Vivian, 100, 109, 209
Bray, Robyn, 133
Bray, Shannon, 133
*British North America Act*, 56
Brossard, Liboire, ("Lee"), 107, 119, 125, 195, 209
Buckland, Theresa Jill, 63, 91, 215
Buick, Lorne, 24, 129, 150, 175
Bulent + Lina Dance Studio, 121, 150, 176
Bulent, Karabagli, 176
Caledon, Town of, 157, 159, 167, 211
Calgary & District Square and Round Dancers Association, 138
Calgary International Salsa Congress, 143
Campanelli, Sandra, 24, 119, 144, 195
Canada Council for the Arts, 79, 94, 128, 136, 139, 216, 218, 222
Canada Dance Mapping, 79, 94, 139, 216, 222
Canada Salsa & Bachata Congress, 143, 144
Canadian Dance and Dance Sport Council, 142
Canadian Dance Teachers' Association (CDTA), 139, 141, 149
Canadian DanceSport, 46, 139, 141, 216
Canadian Olde Tyme Square Dance Association, 88, 153, 154
Canadian Square & Round Dance Society, 86, 153, 154
Cardinal, Sylvain, 163, 186
Carleton, Alexander, 115, 122, 209
Caron, Shirley, 24, 175, 180
Carroll, Lewis, 98
Carrothers, C.C., 71
Casa Loma, 72
Castillo-Mariqueo, Lidia, 135, 137, 218
Cayton-Tang, Beverley, 142, 183, 192
CDA Dance Academy, 111
CDTA, 140
Celia Franca Centre, 133
Central Christian Church, 134
Chan, Lina, 150, 176
Chance Dance Centre, 130, 182

Chandarana, Nina, 24, 110, 112, 124
Charlottetown Conference, 57
Chen, Peter, 142, 179
Cheng, Fred, 164, 209
Cheung, Ying, 98, 99, 209
Chic de la Danse, 150
Chirca, Cristina, 107, 113, 123, 209
Chow, Juliana, 24, 99, 163, 209
Chu, Angela, 142
churches
    Campbellites, 52
    Church of England, 50
    Irvingites, 52
    Mennonites, 52
    Methodist, 50, 52, 53, 61, 219
    Mormons, 52
City Dance Corps, 151, 176, 191
City of Barrie Hall, 128
Clark, Larry, 114, 126, 167, 209
Clément, Véronique, 84
CM Cha Cha Cha Dance Studio, 142, 182, 191
Coles, Mercy Anne, 57, 61, 221
Collier, Clinton, 25
colony of Canada, 35, 57, 91
Cooke, Maude C. (etiquette), 51, 60, 216
Cooper, Lexi, 128
Corfan, H.H., 70
Count Basie, 72
COVID-19, 18, 40, 83, 84, 91, 95, 97, 98, 99, 122, 126, 127, 128, 133, 138, 139, 163, 165, 219
Craig, Gerald M. (historian), 217
Crisp, Freda, 217
Crossley, H.T. (against dancing), 217
cross-selling, 165
Crystal Ballroom Studio, 142
cuers, 139, 152
Cuesteps Round Dance Club, 40, 217
Daccord, Ruth, 167
Dahm, Dorothy, 43, 59, 217
Dance Art Studio, 118
Dance Class for People Living with Parkinson's, 133
Dance Club Blue Silver, 183
Dance Education Network (Québec), 84
Dance for Parkinson's Network Canada

(DFPNC), 132
Dance for PD, 132, 133, 134
*Dance Hall* (movie), 69
dance venues
  Alexandra, 73
  Casa Loma (Toronto), 72
  Palace Pier (Toronto), 72
  Palais Royale (Toronto), 72
  Rebekah Lodge (Lethbridge), 74
dance/movement therapy (DMT), 134
Dance4U, 189
*dancemasters*, 47
dancers, East European, 79
dances
  lindy hop, 80, 115, 122
  paso doble, 135
  rumba, 80
dances, European, Afro-Latin, North American
  black bottom, 68
  bourree, 43
  bump, 77
  cabbage patch, 77
  Celtic, 32
  cha-cha, 43, 67, 80, 109, 119, 159
  Charleston, 68, 69, 80, 164
  checken scratch, 25
  chicken, 77
  clogging, 151
  contra, 151
  contradanse, 39, 43, 151
  cotillion, 26, 43, 49
  dog, 77
  frug, 77
  funky chicken, 77
  grizzly bear, 25
  hustle, 77
  mashed potato, 77
  moonwalk, 77
  pony, 77
  roger rabbit, 77
  running man, 77
  shake, 77
  snake, 77
  swim, 77
  tea, 35, 163
  turkey trot, 25, 64
  twist, 77, 80
  waltz, 21, 43, 47, 49, 52, 60, 66, 67, 69, 70, 81, 93, 109, 114, 119, 220
  West Coast swing, 80, 98, 115, 122
  YMCA, 77
dances, indigenous
  braid bundle, 35
  fancy shawl, 33
  grass, 33
  jingle dress, 33
  men's traditional, 33
  prairie chicken, 33
  round, 33
DanceScape, 142, 183, 192
DanceSport BC, 99
dancing
  18th century, 42
  19th century, 42
  20th century, 62
  ceremonial, 17, 31, 36, 50
  daytime, 55
  elite, 26, 38, 46, 47, 48, 58, 163
  English Style, 81
  food (hunting for), 31
  group, 31, 50
  help from technology, 68
  hotels. See hotels (for dancing)
  line dancing, 111, 151
  manners, 46, 53, 60, 216
  middle class, 45, 47, 72
  powwow, 33
  pre-Confederation, 38
  Prohibition (during), 69, 75
  regalia, 31, 33, 34, 39, 222
  solo, 31
  speakeasies, 69
  spiritual, 17, 31, 40, 221
Dancing for Dessert, 19, 140, 174, 179, 189
dancing forms (shifts in), 42
Dancing with Parkinson's, 213
*Dancing with the Stars*, 83, 97, 168, 170, 171
Davis, Charles Freeman, 70
De Torres, Angelo, 144, 194
deejays, 21, 152
Delgado, Rene, 24, 144
Delta Dance, 140, 179
Dett, R. Nathaniel (composer), 64

Dina, Christina Amalia, 118
Dina, Cristina Amalia, 141
Dobrynin, Alex, 105
Dobrynina, Maria, 105, 167, 211
Dominion of Canada, 56, 58
Doolittle, Lisa, 73
Doyle, Irene, 134
Drinking and Dancing venues, 76
Dubé, Michel, 90, 141, 181, 209
Duchess of Connaught, 67
Dyke, Eleanor, 24, 103, 209
E&R Ballroom Studio, 87
Earhart, Gammon, 134
East Gwillimbury, Town of, 104, 109, 157, 159, 160, 169, 184, 192, 211
Eckstein, Willie, 64
Edgett Dance and Wellness, 141
Edmonton, City of, 74, 140, 157, 159, 160
Edney, Sue, 168
EKOS Research Associates Inc, 94, 218
Elite Dance Studio, 140, 178
Epprecht, Mandy, 18, 24, 88, 141, 163, 164, 166, 185, 193, 209
Etchemins, 35
Evaluation Centre for Complex Health Interventions (TECCHI), 137
Evans, Jim, 105, 116, 125, 209
Evelyn, Gregory, 97, 210
fiddle music, 32, 98
Firth, Edith G., 45
Fisher, James, 153
Flatman, Donna, 168
Foley, Brooklyn, 168
Foley, Rosemarie, 24
FollowMaxFomin, 141, 187
Fomin, Max, 141
Forbes-Anderson, Faye, 23, 211
Forde, Jim, 168
Franks, David, 106, 119, 209
Fred Astaire, 82, 184, 192
Fredericton Swing Dance, 115, 122
Fulton, Mary, 83, 186, 210
Fung, Tony, 142, 179
Gibzey, William, 168
Giménez-Llort, Lydia, 135, 137, 218
Goh, Patricia, 163, 183
Gonzalez, Marina, 87, 174

Gowder, Paul, 33
Graham, Trena, 24, 122, 144, 181, 190
Great Depression, 62, 71, 213
Great Hall, 163
Greenhill, Judy, 210
Gronau, Jim, 144
Gurnon, Stephanie, 144
Halifax, City of, 56, 72, 90, 95, 108, 114, 115, 122, 126, 129, 135, 137, 141, 144, 150, 157, 167, 171, 175, 181, 190, 211, 215
Hall, Larry, 163, 184
Happily Ever Active, 130
Harasymchuk, Dennis, 89, 182, 191
Harbourfront, 112
Henssen, Jeff, 3
Hill, Colin, 135, 137
Hill, Valery, 135, 210
Hirose, Regan, 143
Hobbs, Reverend Richard (against dancing), 52
Hoefnagels, Anna (musicologist), 34, 40, 219
Holliday-Tucker, Sandra, 106, 124, 168, 210
Holly, Veronica, 168
hotels (for dancing)
    Château Frontenac, 72
    Empress, 72
    King Edward, 72
    Mount Royal, 72
    Nova Scotia, 72
    Royal York (Fairmont Royal), 72
    Vancouver, 72
    Windsor, 72
Hung, Faye, 142, 179
Hunter, W.J., 53, 61
Huqqullaaqatigiit, 86
Huqqullaaqatigiit (drumming), 53
hurdy-gurdy (musical instrument), 37
*I Lost My Gig*, 139, 219
Ieropoli, Adriano, 144
Imperial Society of Teachers of Dancing, 70, 141, 142
Inuvialuit, 32, 219
Jackson, Micheal, 77
Jazz Age, 68
JC Dance Co, 163, 179

Jestin, Jerry, 23, 152, 211
Kallmann, Helmut Max (musicologist), 36, 38, 40, 41, 219
Kanyo, Ginette, 24
Kanyo, John, 24, 103
Karakulak, Deniz, 138
Kazi, Omar, 111, 118, 168, 209
Keating, Nella, 168
Keating, Patrick, 103, 169
Kelowna Ballroom, 96, 179, 189
Kimball, Rob and Cathy, 82
King Township, 110
King's daughters, 38
Kitchener, City of, 157, 159, 161, 164, 176, 184, 185, 186, 192, 201, 211
kizomba, 25, 87, 110, 120, 125
Kostov, Stilian, 163, 185
Krzyszkowksi, Derek, 163
KV Ballroom Dancing studio, 90
Kwakwaka'wakw, 52
Lacroix, Dominic, 140, 178
Lajoie, Shirley, 210
Lam, Patricia, 110, 120, 125, 211
Latin Energy Dance Company, 144, 176, 192
Latin Groove, 107, 113, 119, 123, 125
Latin Groove Dance & Fitness, 144, 195
Lebedev, Anton, 187
Lee, Karen, 133, 181, 191
Lee, Kelvin, 169
Lee, Phil, 163, 183
Leong, Ivan, 113, 120, 210
Leung, Santha, 24, 113, 120, 210
Liang, Sarah, 142, 179
Little, Dean, 24, 103, 209
Littlefair, Dave, 152
Loomis, John, 117, 210
Lopez, Ana Karen, 143, 190
Lopez, Leonardo, 143, 190
Lord Aberdeen, 58
Lotta Boucher School of Dancing, Edmonton (1922), 75
Lubberts, Dale, 169
Lubberts, Jelies J., 169
Lusic, Bobbi, 149, 174
Lusic, Patricia, 149, 174
Luttrell, Janis, 23, 161, 211

Ma, Mark, 142, 179
Mackie, Flori, 24, 169
Mainstream & Plus, 109
Malleck, Dan (historian), 220
Malnig, Julie, 49, 60
Mandy's Dance, 18, 88, 123, 141, 185, 193
Maple Ridge, City of, 157, 159, 161, 198, 211
Marasigan, Joel, 87, 163, 179
Maria, Ishbel, 58
Maritime Callers and Cuers Association, 153
Mark Morris Dance Company, 131
Massoud, Samia, 87, 143, 145, 189
Mastrandrea, Pat, 111, 121, 169, 210
McClure United Church, 133
McCombs, Barrie, 138
McCormack, Eric, 154, 210
McDonald, Anne (author), 57
McEllistrum, Kyra, 164
McIntosh, Andrew, 140, 174, 179, 189
McKay, Louise, 97, 98, 116, 211
McKinley, Patricia, 134
McMains, Juliet, 46, 59, 63, 65, 67, 81, 82, 91, 92, 93, 94, 221
Meinecke, Alice, 98, 124, 210
Mercado-Alatrista, Wolfgang, 150
Merchandise, 165
Métis, 31, 32, 33, 39, 45
Meyer, Merv, 108, 210
Meyer, Sandy-Gregson, 108
Mi'kmaqs, 35, 36
Michel & Company, 90, 95, 141, 181
Millet, Cheryl, 169
*milonga*, 115, 125, 126
Mina, Abby, 144, 181, 191
Mitchell, Brenton, 141, 181
MonTango, 150
Montreal Salsa Convention, 143
Monty, Gabriel, 149
*Moose Jaw Herald Times*, 109
Morina, Vahide, 114, 122, 126, 210
Movers and Shakers group, (P.E.I.), 134
Mulrooney, Angela, 149, 188
Muretov, Sergey, 130, 182
Murgatroyd, Steve, 163, 185
Nader, Karen Abi, 25

Naeem, Uzma, 169
Najarian, Apo, 25
Nakamura, Maryrose, 170, 211
Naranjo, Oscar, 145, 193
National Ballet School, 132, 133
Natsvlichvili, Tinko, 89
naturopathic doctor, 117
Nelson, Steve, 24, 142, 163, 184, 198, 210
Nest Building, 163
Newmarket
    2015-2025 Recreation Playbook, 155
    Cultural Master Plan, 155
    Seniors' Meeting Place, 111
Newmarket, Town of, 105, 106, 111, 119, 121, 124, 130, 155, 157, 159, 161, 167, 168, 169, 170, 171, 182, 194, 201, 211
Nichol, Estelle, 176
North Vancouver, City of, 133, 155, 157, 211
Novaera Productions, 144
Ogina, Julia, 87
Okazawa, Tadahiro, 97, 116, 211
Old Mill, 119
Ontario Brain Institute Evaluation Support Program, 137
Ontario Hydro, 103
*Ontario Regulation 546/20*, 86
Ontario Trillium Foundation, 130
orchestras
    Dave Mills, 74
    Duke Ellington, 68, 74, 93, 213
    Mart Kenney and His Western Gentlemen, 74
    Sunny Fry, 74
Order of Good Cheer, 37
Outevsky, David, 77, 79, 94, 221
Panacci, Dianne, 110
Panacci, Dominic, 110, 170, 210
Pan-American games, 150
pandemic, 18, 40, 83, 84, 86, 87, 88, 89, 90, 91, 96, 97, 98, 99, 118, 119, 121, 122, 123, 126, 127, 133, 135, 138, 154, 155, 163, 165, 166, *See* COVID-19
Parkinson Canada, 132
Parkinson's disease, 26, 129, 130, 131, 132, 133, 135, 136, 137, 150, 215
parkinsonism, 132
Parks, Paul, 135, 137
Parks, Theresa, 210
Paton-Evans, Karen, 105, 116, 125
Penobscots, 35
Pointe Claire, City of, 203
Potlatch, 60, 218
Price, Ralph, 24, 88, 153, 154, 155, 210
Price, Sandy, 153
Prince of Wales (Albert Edward), 55, 61, 222
Pro-Am World Salsa Championships, 143
Pugliese, Francesco, 24, 170
Pytlik, George, 83, 94, 179
Pytlik, Wendy, 140, 179
Québec Conference, 56
Queen Victoria
    effect on dancing, 46, 50, 58, 63
Radford, Ian (historian), 56
Ramsay, Janis, 222
Rancon, Harold, 143
Reid, Darren, 170
Reid, Trisha, 170
RHR Latin Dance Company, 143
Rhythm & Motion Dance Studio, 150, 177, 193
Rideau Hall, 58, 68, 92
Roaring Twenties, 25
Robichaud, Sarah, 131
Robinson, Amanda, 31
Robson Square Summer Dance Series, 99
Robson, Jesse, 130
Romaire, Delphine, 140
Rough 'n' Ready Spinsters' Club, 71
Royal Canadian Yacht Club, 55
Royal City Squares, 153, 202
Roy-Pleau, Raymonde, 170
Rudzik, Magda, 24, 140, 174, 179, 189
Russell, Bill, 24, 154, 155
Russo, Louise, 130
Ryder, Brenda, 152
Sadowska, Elizabeth, 24, 117, 121, 150, 185
Sage, Jessica, 87, 143, 145, 189
Saint-Bruno, 107

Saiyan, Aleksander, 24, 89, 112, 143, 194, 210
Salmon Arm, City of, 158, 162, 168, 197, 198, 212
Salon Tango Championship, 149
Salsa Explosion Dance Company, 88, 95
Salsa on St. Clair, 99
*salseros(as)*, 97, 144
San Tropez Dance Centre, 89, 195
*Sandra & the Latin Groove Band*, 144
Saskatchewan Square & Round Dance Federation, 100, 109
Saskatoon, 87, 100, 133, 177, 187, 195, 203, 205
Sato, Leo, 24, 87, 95, 116, 149, 174
Scali, Samantha, 144
Sedman, Bud, 152, 210
Shaheen, Qasira, 170
Shepherd, Andrea, 150
Sherren, Anna, 152
Sherren, Roger, 152
Shih-Marasigan, Clara, 163
Shum, Gerry, 170
Simcoe Muskoka District Health Unit, 128
Simcoe, Elizabeth Posthuma, 44
Slone, Isabel B., 96
Smith, Larratt William Violet, 48
Solomon, Corey, 87, 143, 145, 189, 210
Sommer, Martina, 24, 129, 150, 175
Square and Round Dance Instructors Association of Alberta, 152
Square Dance Calgary, 138
Square Dancing, 153
Srigley, Katrina, 71, 93, 222
Stanfield, Barry, 107, 210
Stanfield, Esther, 107, 210
Stardust Dance Productions, 121
Stay, Vanessa, 144
Stefaniak, John, 171
Steps Dance Studio, 144, 185, 194
Stevens, Lys, 80, 94, 222
Stone, Kathryn, 108, 210
Stradling, Cindy, 118, 121, 210
Straight, Megan Walter, 24, 133, 134
Szymczak, Monika, 120, 125, 210
Tan, Timothy, 123

*tanda*, 97
Tang, Robert, 142, 183, 192
Tango8Fest, 151
TangoBug studio, 149
*tangueros(as)*, 89, 97
Tea & Tango, 26, 129, 130, 135, 136, 150, 175
tea room 18th century, 49
Ten Dance competition, 140, 141
Ternan, Dianne, 106, 119, 209
*The Spanish Dancer (movie)*, 69
Theyyil, Ashika, 171
Thibault, Richard, 142, 163, 185
Thompson Valley Stars, 108, 198
Thompson-Shuswap Square & Round Dance Association, 109
Thorburn, Chris, 96, 128, 179, 189, 223
Toronto Dance Professionals, 138, 186
Toronto Dance Salsa, 89, 95, 110, 112, 143, 194, 223
*Toronto Life*, 96, 224
Toronto square dance festival, 98
Toronto Tango Festival, 149
*Toronto World*, 70, 93, 214, 224
Torres, Giovanni, 145
Tory, John, 85
Tran, Carlo, 182
Tran, Monica, 182
Trenas Studio, 144
Trianon Ballroom, 73, 74, 93, 213
Tucker, Silas ("Sie"), 106, 124, 171
Tulk, Janice E, 223
University of British Columbia (UBC) Dance Club, 95, 98, 223
gala ball, 98
University of Waterloo Ballroom & Latin, 164
UW Swing Club, 164
Val-des-Monts, 158, 160, 162, 212
Vallerand, Francois, 88
Vallerand, Melody, 88, 105
Valvasori, Basil, 81
Vance, Daniela, 171
Vancity International Salsa Bachata Kizomba Festival, 143
Vanderaa, Martin, 108, 127, 210
Vanderaa, Vaunda, 108, 127
Vasarhelyi, Susan, 171

Veloso, Issa, 171
Vetesse, Marla, 163
Victoria Park Community Centre, 105
Viola, Charles J., 70
W., Andria, 117, 118, 122, 171, 210
Waite, P.B., 56, 61, 223
Wallace, James (journalist), 55, 61, 223
Warwick, William (dance publisher), 50, 51, 60, 223
Washington University, 134
Wason, Janet, 58, 61, 223
West-Way Club, 86, 88, 95, 106, 117
Wet'suwet'en hereditary chiefs, 215
Wheel Dance, 130
Whitchurch-Stouffville, Town of, 158, 160, 163, 212
White, Justin, 90, 186
White, Marjorie, 24, 90, 164, 186
Whyte, Jean, 70
Willems, Jacinta, 104, 117, 121, 211
Windsor, City of, 72, 76, 157, 160, 162, 177, 182, 184, 212
Wong, Andy, 142, 180
Wong, Wendy, 180
Wong, Zillion, 87, 142, 179
World Bachata Championship, 145
World Latin Dance Cup, 144
World Salsa Federation, 141
World Tango Championship, 149
Xie, Laurie, 142, 179
Yavorskay, Luiza, 171
*Yes I Dance* survey, 139
You, Two, Can Tango dance studio, 129
Young, Peter (historian), 72
Zalvalna, Julia, 130
Zhang, Linda, 142, 179
zumba, 110

www.ingramcontent.com/pod-product-compliance
Lightning Source LLC
LaVergne TN
LVHW021810060526
838201LV00058B/3320